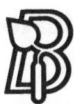

Milestones in Drug Therapy
MDT

Series Editors

Prof. Dr. Michael J. Parnham
PLIVA
Research Institute
Prilaz baruna Filipovica 25
10000 Zagreb
Croatia

Prof. Dr. J. Bruinvels
INFARM
Sweelincklaan 75
NL-3723 JC Bilthoven
The Netherlands

ACE Inhibitors

Edited by P. D'Orléans-Juste and G. E. Plante

Birkhäuser Verlag
Basel . Boston . Berlin

Editors

Pedro D'Orléans-Juste
Gérard E. Plante
Department of Pharmacology
Institute of Pharmacology of Sherbrooke
Medical School
Sherbrooke University
Sherbrooke, PQ
Canada J1H-5N4

Library of Congress Cataloging-in-Publication Data
ACE inhibitors / edited by P. D'Orléans-Juste and G.E. Plante.
   p. ; cm. — (Milestones in drug therapy)
 Includes bibliographical references and index.
 ISBN 978-3-0348-7581-3
  1. Angiotensin converting enzyme—Inhibitors. I. D'Orléans-Juste, P. (Pedro), 1957-
 II. Plante, G. E. (Gérard E.) III. Series.
 [DNLM: 1. Angiotensin-Converting Enzyme Inhibitors—pharmacology.
 2. Angiotensin-Converting Enzyme Inhibitors—therapeutic use. 3. Cardiovascular
 Diseases—drug therapy. QV 150 A1727 2001]
 RC684.A53 A25 2001
 616.1'061–dc21

Deutsche Bibliothek Cataloging-in-Publication Data
ACE inhibitors / ed. by P. D'Orléans-Juste and G. E. Plante. - Basel ; Boston ; Berlin :
Birkhäuser, 2001
   (Milestones in drug therapy)

 ISBN 978-3-0348-7581-3   ISBN 978-3-0348-7579-0 (eBook)
 DOI 10.1007/978-3-0348-7579-0

Table of contents

List of contributors

Albert Adam, Faculté de pharmacie, Université de Montréal, 2900 Boulevard Edouard-Montpetit, Montréal, QC, H3C 3J7, Canada; e-mail: adama@pharm.umontreal.ca

Athanase Benetos, Unité INSERM 337, Institut des cordeliers+, 15 rue de l'école de médicine, 75006 Paris, France; e-mail: benetos@ccr.jussieu.fr

Charles Blais Jr., Faculté de pharmacie, Université de Montréal, 2900 Boulevard Edouard-Montpetit, Montréal, QC, H3C 3J7, Canada; e-mail: ...

Harry A.J. Struijker Boudier, Department of Pharmacology, University of Limburg, 6200 MD-Maastricht, The Netherlands; e-mail: H.StruijkerBoudier@Farmaco.UNIMAAS.NL

John D. Catravas, Vascular Biology Center, Medical College of Georgia, Augusta, GA 30912-2500, USA; e-mail: jcatrava@mail.mcg.edu

Jacques de Champlain, Department of Physiology, Faculty of Medicine, Université de Montéal, P.O. Box 6128, Station Centre-Ville, Montréal (Québec) H3C 3J7, Canada; e-mail: dechampj@physio.umontreal.ca

Mark E. Cooper, Department of Medicine, Austin & Repatriation Medical Centre (Repatriation Campus), West Heidelberg, Victoria 3081, Australia; e-mail: cooper@austin.unimelb.edu.au

Pedro D'Orléans-Juste, Department of Pharmacology, Institute of Pharmacology of Sherbrooke, Medical School, Sherbrooke University, Sherbrooke, PQ, Canada J1H-5N4; e-mail: labpdj@courrier.usherb.ca

Cynthia A. Fink, Metabolic and Cardiovascular Diseases Research, Novartis Biomedical Research Institute, Summit, New Jersey 07901, USA; e-mail: cynthia.fink@pharma.novartis.com

Eve-Reine Gagné, Department of Medicine (Nephrology), University of Sherbrooke, Sherbrooke (Québec), Canada; e-mail: ergagne@courrier.usherb.ca

Haralambos Gavras, Hypertension and Atherosclerosis Section, Boston University School of Medicine, 715 Albany Street, Boston, MA 02118, USA; e-mail: hgavras@bu.edu

Irene Gavras, Hypertension and Atherosclerosis Section, Boston University School of Medicine, 715 Albany Street, Boston, MA 02118, USA; e-mail: igavras@bu.edu

Venkat Gopalakrishnan, Department of Pharmacology, College of Medicine, University of Saskatchewan, Saskatoon SK, Canada S7N 5E5; e-mail: gopal@sask.usask.ca

Rob L. Hopfner, Department of Pharmacology, College of Medicine, University of Saskatchewan, Saskatoon SK, Canada S7N 5E5; e-mail: rhopfner@gsb.uchicago.edu

Malika Lajemi, Unité INSERM 337, Institut des cordelier, 15 rue de l'école de médicine, 75006 Paris, France; e-mail: lajemi@ccr.jussieu.fr

Maxime Lamarre-Cliche, Department of Medicine, Internal Medicine Service,

Centre Hospitalier de l'Université de Montréal, Hôtel-Dieu, 3840, Saint-Urbain Street, Montréal, Québec H2W 1T8, Canada

Pierre Larochelle, Department of Medicine, Internal Medicine Service, Centre Hospitalier de l'Université de Montréal, Hôtel-Dieu, 3840, Saint-Urbain Street, Montréal, Québec H2W 1T8, Canada; e-mail: pierre.larochelle@umontreal.ca

Wolfgang Linz, Aventis Pharma Deutschland GmbH, Cardiovascular Disease Group, Building H821, 65926 Frankfurt/Main, Germany; e-mail: Wolfgang.Linz@aventis.com

Gérard M. London, Service de Néphrologie, Centre Hospitalier F. H. Manhes, 91700 Fleury Mérogis, France; e-mail: glondon@club-internet.fr

François Marceau, Centre Hospitalier Universitaire de Québec, Centre de Recherche du Pavillon L'Hôtel-Dieu de Québec, Québec, QC, G1R 2J6, Canada

J. Robert McNeill, Department of Pharmacology, College of Medicine, University of Saskatchewan, Saskatoon SK, Canada S7N 5E5; e-mail: Robert.McNeill@usask.ca

Gérard E. Plante, Departments of Medicine (Nephrology), Physiology and Pharmacology, Institute of Pharmacology, University of Sherbrooke, Sherbrooke (Québec), Canada; e-mail: geplante@courrier.usherb.ca

Tewfik Nawar, Departments of Medicine (Nephrology), University of Sherbrooke, Sherbrooke (Québec), Canada; e-mail: t.nawar@courrier.usherb.ca

Stylianos E. Orfanos, Department of Critical Care and Pulmonary Medicine, Evangelismos Hospital, University of Athens Medical School, Athens, Greece; e-mail: stelmar@ath.forthnet.gr

Michel E. Safar, Service de Médecine 1, Hôpital Broussais, 96, rue Didot, 75674 Paris, France; e-mail: michel.safar@brs.ap-hop-paris.fr

Bernward A. Schölkens, Aventis Pharma Deutschland GmbH, Disease Groups Research, Building H821, 65926 Frankfurt/Main, Germany; e-mail: bernward.schoelkens@aventis.com

Raymonde Turcotte, Departments of Medicine (Nephrology), Physiology and Pharmacology, Institute of Pharmacology, University of Sherbrooke, Sherbrooke (Québec), Canada

Luc M. A. B. Van Bortel, Department of Pharmacology, University of Limburg, 6200 MD-Maastricht, The Netherlands; e-mail: luc.vanbortel@rug.ac.be

John R. Vane, The William Harvey Research Foundation, Charterhouse Square, London EC1M 6BQ, UK; e-mail: c.l.measures@mds.qmw.ac.uk

Gabriele Wiemer, Aventis Pharma Deutschland GmbH, Cardiovascular Disease Group, Building H821, 65926 Frankfurt/Main, Germany; e-mail: gabriele.wiemer@aventis.com

Paulus Wohlfart, Aventis Pharma Deutschland GmbH, Cardiovascular Disease Group, Building H821, 65926 Frankfurt/Main, Germany; e-mail: paulus.wohlfart@aventis.com

Linhua Zou, Vascular Biology Center, Medical College of Georgia, Augusta, GA 30912-2500, USA; e-mail: lzou@mail.mcg.edu

Preface

Angiotensin converting enzyme inhibitors (ACEI) represent the first class of antihypertensive agents that was designed and developed on the basis of a well-defined physiopathological axis of arterial hypertension, a vascular disorder that is now becoming one of the major causes of morbidity/mortality, not only in developed societies but also in the highly populated developing countries [1].

CAPTOPRIL, the prototype of the "PRIL" family, which now comprises more than 40 molecule-species, was quite hazardous and the clinical development almost failed when serious side-effects were reported in an alarmist fashion in reputable scientific journals, such as the *New England Journal of Medicine* and *Lancet*. Squibb & Sons came very close to withdrawing CAPTOPRIL from clinical investigation [2].

However, after re-examination of the data obtained from different categories of patients and appropriate dose-adjustments, the clinical use of CAPTOPRIL turned out to be revolutionary. The prototype, as well as other members of the "PRIL" family became the starting point for numerous basic and clinical research programs, focusing on the interactions of ACEI with the kinin, endothelin, and nitric oxide systems, and the contribution of the receptors for AT_1, AT_2, bradykinin B_1 and B_2, ET_A and ET_B to the pharmacological actions of the respective peptides. This research activity led to the development of new pharmacological agents, such as the angiotensin receptor antagonists and, more recently, the neutral endopeptidase inhibitors. In the near future, bradykinin receptor antagonists also will be available to modulate ACEI pharmacological actions.

Surprisingly, despite the tremendous pharmaceutical development in this important area of medicine, there have been fewer than half a dozen comprehensive textbooks on the basic and clinical sciences related to the field of ACEIs. Therefore, we felt that the publication of the present book was justified by the dramatic evolution of knowledge in the field of ACEI over the past decade.

The Nobel Prize recipient John R. Vane generously agreed to introduce this book on ACEI by reviewing the history of this unique class of antihypertensive drugs. The following chapters will present in two different sections basic science knowledge and clinical aspects related to ACEI. The relationship between ACEI and bradykinin metabolism and the interactions between ACEI, endothelin pathway, nitric oxide production, and neutral endopeptidase also will be examined in four different chapters. The latter will be followed by pharmacological aspects of ACEI, including the tissue-specificity mode of actions, the genetic basis of the clinical response of patients in relation to the risk of arterial disease. Important and relatively ignored actions of ACEI on the central and peripheral autonomic nervous systems will be discussed in two additional chapters. In one of these, the poorly known effect of ACEI on thirst and salt appetite examined in hypertensive subjects also will be presented.

The mechanisms involved in target organ damage that is responsible for morbidity and mortality observed in most vascular diseases, including arterial hypertension, diabetes mellitus, and heart and renal failure, will be re-examined on revisited aspects of the microcirculation networks and the potent effects of ACEI on these poorly examined segments of the vasculature and presented in a separate chapter, which introduces the clinical component of the book. Evaluative and epidemiological approaches of ACEI therapy, including recent comparative guidelines in arterial hypertension, will be presented. The use of ACEI in the treatment of heart failure and the critical interest of the "PRILs" in the prevention and treatment of diabetes mellitus renal complications will be reviewed. Finally, the effect of ACEI on large artery structure and function in arterial hypertension will be presented by a group of European scientists actively involved in that critical area of vascular research, perhaps representing the key answer to senescence.

The final word is to express our sincere gratitude to all of the contributors to this monograph on ACE inhibitors for sharing with the readers their internationally recognised expertise.

Pedro D'Orléans-Juste
Gérard E. Plante

1   Guidelines Subcommittee (WHO-ISH) World Health organization-International Society for Hypertension (1999) Guidelines for the management of Hypertension. *J Hypertension* 17:151–183
2   Plante GE (2000) Traitement sans bogue de l'hypertension artérielle au nouveau millénaire. Nouvelle pharmacologie du système rénine-angiotensine. *Médecine Sciences* 16: 14–17

ACE Inhibitors
ed. by P. D'Orléans-Juste and G.E. Plante
© 2001 Birkhäuser Verlag/Switzerland

The history of inhibitors of angiotensin converting enzyme

John R. Vane

The William Harvey Research Foundation, Charterhouse Square, London EC1M 6BQ, UK

Just over 100 years ago Felix Hoffman synthesised acetylsalicylic acid, which was marketed as Aspirin by the Bayer Company. It is now selling more than 45,000 tonnes per year. The story of the aspirin-like drugs [1] is a fascinating one, in which our discovery that they inhibit the formation of prostaglandins (PGs) [2] was a key stepping stone in its development. The enzyme involved is cyclooxygenase (COX) and we now know that there are at least two isozymes, COX-1 and COX-2. Now we have selective COX-2 inhibitors, which have the promise of being excellent anti-inflammatory drugs without the side effects on the stomach [3].

In this chapter I will relate our involvement in a different field, that of the renin angiotensin system. At about the same time that Felix Hoffmann was synthesising aspirin, Tigerstedt and Bergman in 1898 [4] found that crude saline extracts of the kidney contained a long-acting pressor substance, which they named renin. This fundamental observation led, over the next 100 years, to the elucidation of the complex renin angiotensin system involving such famous names as Goldblatt, Braun-Menendez, Bumpus and Page, Skeggs, Gross, Peart and many others. We became involved in the late 1960s and our research work led to the discovery of angiotensin converting enzyme inhibitors.

First, what is the renin angiotensin system? Renin is an enzyme stored by the granular juxtaglomerular cells that lie in the walls of the afferent arterioles as they enter the glomerulae. Renin is a protease, its principle natural substrate being the circulating $\alpha2$-globulin called angiotensinogen. The active form of renin is a glycoprotein that contains 340 amino acids. This is synthesised as a pre-pro enzyme of 460 amino acids but is processed to pro-renin a mature, but inactive form of the protein.

There are numerous ways of activating the secretion of renin from the kidney into the bloodstream, where it chops the decapeptide angiotensin-1 from the aminoterminal end of angiotensinogen, a 452 amino acid plasma protein.

Angiotensin converting enzyme (ACE) is the second enzyme (Fig. 1) in the cascade. Skeggs discovered it in plasma serendipitously in 1956 [5] as the factor responsible for conversion of the inactive decapeptide, angiotensin I, to the

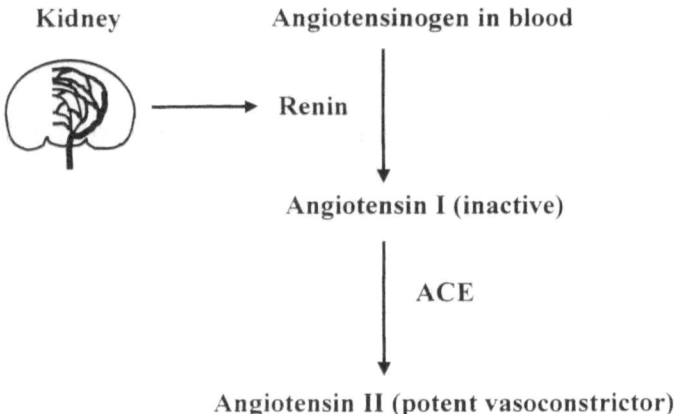

Figure 1. The renin-angiotensin system.

potent pressor octapeptide, angiotensin II. Human ACE contains 1278 amino acid residues and is rather non-specific in that it cleaves dipeptide units from substrates with diverse amino acid sequences, including angiotensin I and bradykinin.

When we started our work in the field it was assumed that the inactive angiotensin I was converted to the potent pressor substance angiotensin II by ACE in the plasma. This was because when angiotensin I was injected intravenously there was a rapid rise in blood pressure due to the formation of angiotensin II, suggesting that the plasma enzyme was a potent one. We tested this hypothesis using the blood-bathed organ technique [6]. In this method, different isolated organs are superfused continuously with heparinised blood taken at a rate of 10 ml/min from an anaesthetised cat or dog and then returned into the animal intravenously. Over the years we chose a series of different isolated organs which would react differently to endogenous hormones so that we could measure adrenaline by a rat stomach strip and a chick rectum, angiotensin II by a rat colon, bradykinin by a cat jejunum and so on [7].

We wanted to measure the rate of conversion of angiotensin I to angiotensin II in blood so we used an incubating circuit into which we could infuse either substance with a defined delay of anything up to three minutes before it reached the assay tissues [8]. We were surprised to find that there was little or no conversion of angiotensin I to angiotensin II in the bloodstream. For instance, there was only 27% conversion of angiotensin I to angiotensin II after 15 s. incubation with blood, 40% after 60 s. and 93% after 180 s. Remembering that a complete circulation time is around 30 s., this is a slow rate of conversion. We, therefore, began to examine infusions of the angiotensins into different parts of the circulation. We found that when infused intravenously, using a rat colon bathed in femoral arterial blood to measure the effects after passage through the pulmonary circulation, there was an increase in activity as

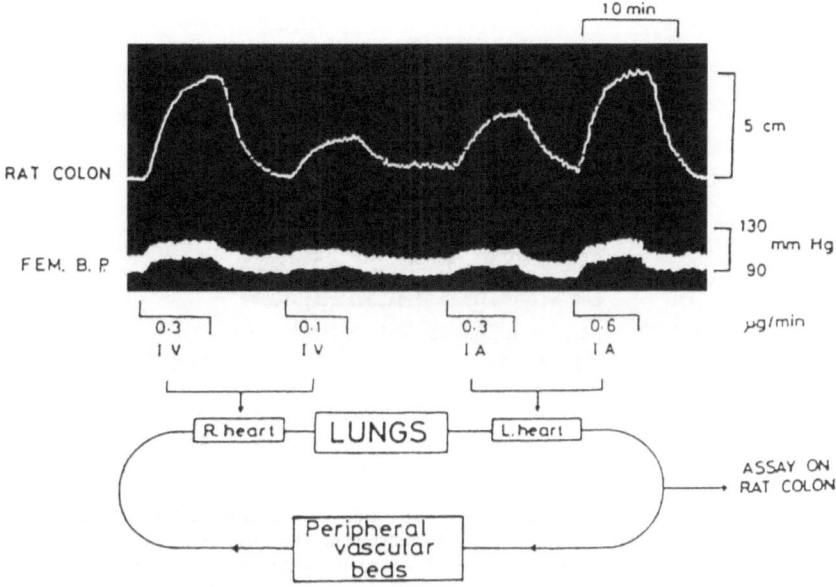

Figure 2. Increase in activity of angiotensin I on passage through the pulmonary circulation *in vivo*. This tracing shows the responses of a rat isolated colon superfused with femoral arterial blood from a dog and the dog's blood pressure. Angiotensin I was infused as shown either into the right ventricle (i.v.) or the ascending aorta (i.a.). Comparing the first and third responses, an infusion of 0.3 µg/min given i.v. was more effective than the same amount infused i.a. The effects of the angiotensin I that had passed through the pulmonary circulation (0.3 µg/min i.v.) were equivalent to those of twice the infusion (0.6 µg/min) given i.a. (from [10] with permission).

the angiotensin I transgressed the lungs (Fig. 2). There was a strong conversion of angiotensin I to angiotensin II in the few seconds it takes to cross the pulmonary circulation. We repeated this experiment in several ways, as well as measuring the lack of conversion of angiotensin I across other vascular beds [8]. To make sure the plasma had no effect on this process, we perfused an isolated lung from a guinea pig with Krebs' solution and found the same conversion, as seen in Figure 3 [9].

Our discovery that ACE largely resided in the pulmonary tissues was an exciting one. We did not know which cell contained ACE but we did speculate that, because bradykinin was also largely inactivated in the pulmonary circulation, ACE and bradykininase may be the same enzyme [10]. Erdos and his colleagues [11] then showed that ACE was identical to kininase II. It was left to Una Ryan et al. [12] to localize the enzyme on the luminal surface of the vascular endothelial cells. There followed an explosion of research on the metabolic function of the lung [7], which turns out to be largely associated with the endothelial cell [13, 14]. This single layer lining of the blood vasculature is responsible, not only for angiotensin conversion, but also for generating the vasodilator and anti-platelet prostacyclin, as well as nitric oxide and

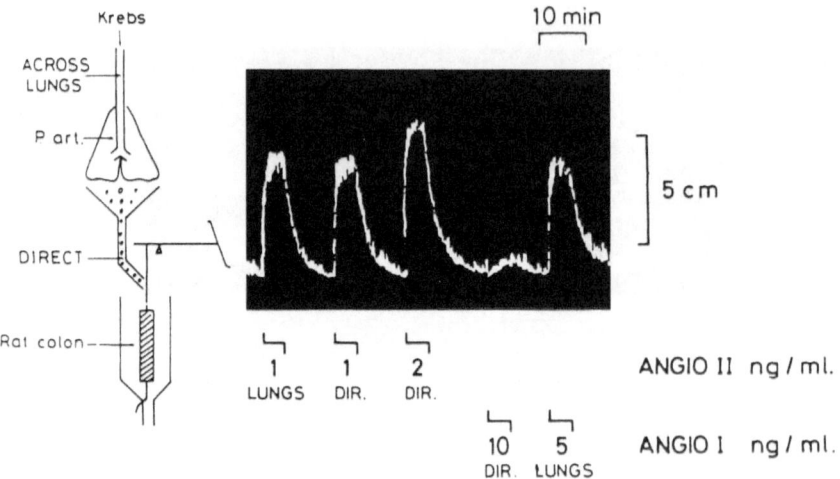

Figure 3. Activation of angiotensin I and free passage of angiotensin II through guinea pig isolated lungs. On the left is a diagram of the experimental arrangement. The lungs were perfused with Krebs' solution via the pulmonary artery and the effluent from the lungs superfused a rat isolated colon. The angiotensins were infused either below the lung (direct), or into the cannula into the pulmonary artery so that they passed through the pulmonary circulation before superfusing the assay tissue. The first two responses show that the activity of angiotensin II is unaffected by passage through the pulmonary circulation; that of angiotensin I (last two responses) greatly increased (5 ng/ml through the lungs causes a much greater response than twice that from infusion, 10 ng/ml, made directly) (from [9] with permission).

endothelin. Furthermore, the endothelium metabolises PGE_1, PGE_2, 5-hydroxy-tryptamine (5-HT), bradykinin and so on [13, 14]. About half of the endothelial cells in the vasculature are in the pulmonary circulation and that is why the lung functions as a metabolic organ.

We were also able to measure the release of angiotensin II by various manipulations of the circulation. For instance, when we inflated a balloon in the aorta of the dog in order to reduce renal arterial pressure, there was an outpouring of renin, which caused generation of angiotensin II [15]. Similarly, when we removed blood from the dog in controlled haemorrhages, there was also generation of angiotensin II followed later by a secretion of adrenaline as shown by relaxation of the rat stomach strip [16]. We were also able to demonstrate an increase of circulating angiotensin II during carotid occlusion in the dog [17].

In the mid 1960s, a Brazilian, Sergio Ferreira, came to work with me as a post-doc. He was carrying in his pocket a dried extract of the venom of the poisonous Brazilian viper Bothrops jararaca. He was trained in the laboratory of Mauricio Roche-e-Silva, who discovered bradykinin in the venom of the snake. Working on the old principle that venom sometimes contained not only noxious substances, but also others that potentiate their effects, Ferreira for his PhD thesis isolated from the venom of the same snake a factor that he called bradykinin potentiating factor or BPF [18].

   Enthusiastically, I suggested to Sergio that he should examine his snake
venom extract on the renin angiotensin system, because we were already
immersed in projects involving angiotensin-I and angiotensin-II. He wanted to
go on with his work on bradykinin, using the blood-bathed organ technique
and being a strong personality, he persuaded me to join him in this work. We
published several interesting papers together on the fate of bradykinin in the
circulation, including the fact that bradykinin was largely inactivated in a single passage through the pulmonary circulation [19–21].
   Eventually, two years later, I persuaded another colleague, Mick Bakhle to
test the snake venom extract on an *in vitro* preparation of angiotensin-converting enzyme and he found it to be a potent inhibitor [22]. We followed this up
on various bioassay preparations and also in the whole animal. As described
above, we had already shown, not only *in vivo* in the dog, but also in isolated
lung preparations, that angiotensin I was largely converted to angiotensin II in
the pulmonary circulation. It was in such preparations that we also showed that
BPF inhibited the conversion of angiotensin I to angiotensin II [23].

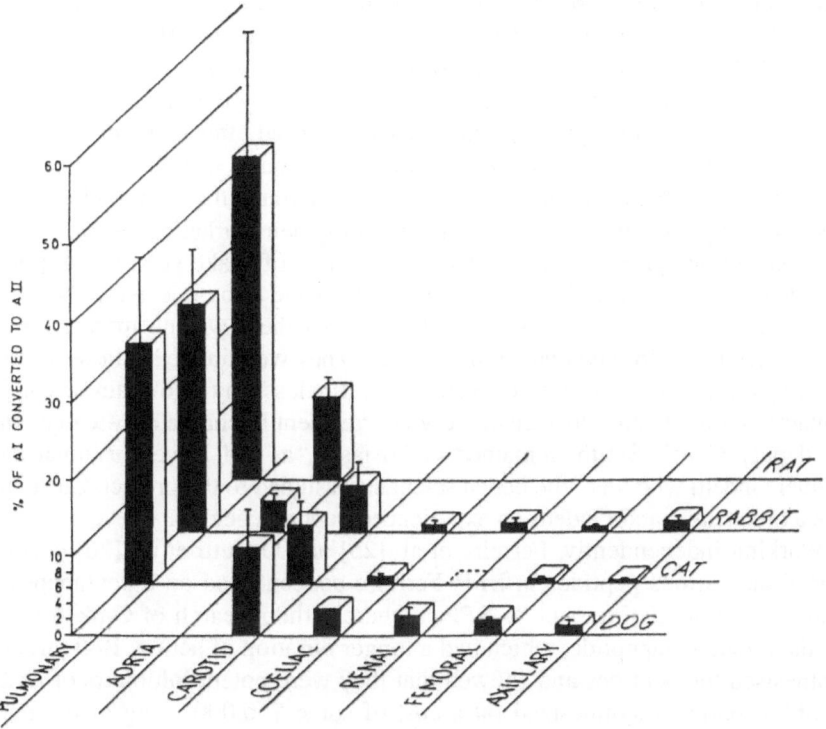

Figure 4. The diagram illustrates the differences in converting enzyme activity shown by arterial strips
from rat, rabbit, cat and dog. The vertical lines at the top of the columns show either the s.e. or the
range when n = 2. Pulmonary arteries showed the highest activity, then rat aorta and then the carotid
arteries. Coeliac, renal, femoral and axillary arteries had little or no activity. The cat renal artery did
not contract to the angiotensins (from [23] with permission).

Interestingly, as shown in Figure 4, the converting enzyme activity in isolated arterial vessel strips varied from vessel to vessel, but not much from species to species. Pulmonary arteries showed the highest activity, then rat aorta and then the carotid arteries. Coeliac, renal, femoral and axillary arteries had little or no activity. In the light of the localisation of ACE on the surface of the endothelial cell, these observations suggest that the levels of ACE vary according to the locality in the circulation.

Much earlier, for my own post-doc experience, I went in 1953 to work at Yale University with Arnold Welch, who had just become the Professor of Pharmacology and I spent two happy years there. By the mid 1960s, he had moved on to become the R&D Director for the pharmaceutical company Squibb in New Jersey and he asked me to act as consultant to them. On one of my early visits I suggested that they should study this snake venom extract, which we then knew to be a mixture of peptides. At that time, no one knew whether angiotensin II formation contributed to high blood pressure. With the isolation, purification and synthesis of one of the peptides from the venom extract, I proposed that they could test whether or not angiotensin II was important in high blood pressure. If it were, then they would have a starting point for a new therapy. Indeed, in parallel work when he returned to Brazil (now convinced that ACE inhibition was important) Ferreira showed in cats that BPF ablated the rise in blood pressure, which was caused by the massive release of renin when the blood supply to a kidney was restored after being clamped for 6 h [24]. BPF also worked in other experimental models of hypertension.

I visited Squibb three times a year and each time found that their initial enthusiasm for the project was waning, mainly because their marketing people did not comprehend that proving a concept with an extract of snake venom could possibly lead to a new drug. Peptides, they argued, have to be injected rather than given orally and they emphatically reiterated that there was no market for an anti-hypertensive drug that had to be injected. They were in the business of selling drugs and not of proving concepts. Nevertheless, my two main scientific contacts at Squibb, Arnold Welch, the Vice-President in charge of research, and his deputy Chuck Smith, remained enthusiastic, as did Dave Cushman and Miguel Ondetti who were the bench scientists assigned to the project. Cushman was a biochemist and Ondetti an experienced peptide chemist.

Working independently, Ferreira et al. [25] and Ondetti et al. [26] characterised the various peptides in BPF. Ferreira concentrated on a pentapeptide, bradykinin potentiating peptide BPP_{5a}, whereas the research of Ondetti et al. led them to a nonapeptide, which had a longer duration of action. Both groups synthesised the peptides and showed that they were potent inhibitors of ACE. Squibb eventually synthesized (at a cost of some $50,000) 1 kg of the nonapeptide, which they called teprotide.

In London, in 1973, we showed [27] that when volunteers were given teprotide intravenously, a bolus injection intravenously of angiotensin I no longer caused a rise in blood pressure through conversion to angiotensin II, so confirming that it was an ACE inhibitor in man.

Squibb also sent a sample to John Laragh in New York, who was one of the leading specialists in the USA in hypertension. He injected it into some of his hypertensive patients and was delighted to find that the blood pressure was reduced [28, 29]. Thus, the concept was proved: angiotensin II was important in hypertension.

In 1973, I left the Royal College of Surgeons to become the R&D Director at the drug company known as Burroughs Wellcome in the States or as the Wellcome Foundation in the UK. I could not continue my relationship with Squibb: higher management cancelled the project, but Dave Cushman and Miguel Ondetti continued to discuss the concept.

The breakthrough came on Wednesday 13th March 1974, when Ondetti and Cushman were discussing a paper describing inhibitors of the enzyme carboxypeptidase [30]. A number of properties of ACE suggested to them that it was an exopeptidase with an active site similar to that of carboxypeptidase-A, presumably including the presence of zinc iron. They reasoned that the major difference between the exopeptidases was that the active site of ACE had evolved to accommodate a dipeptide residue rather than a single amino acid residue as the leaving group for the peptidolytic reaction that is catalysed (Fig. 5). The compound they first made to accommodate this concept was D-2-methylsuccinyl-L-proline. This did indeed inhibit ACE, but it had a disappointingly low activity.

They then found that the D-2-methyl derivative of succinyl-L-proline was about 15 times more potent and were encouraged when it showed oral activity for ACE inhibition in animal experiments. A further breakthrough was achieved when the carboxylate was replaced by a simple sulphhydryl function giving a 2000-fold increase in potency as an inhibitor of ACE [30].

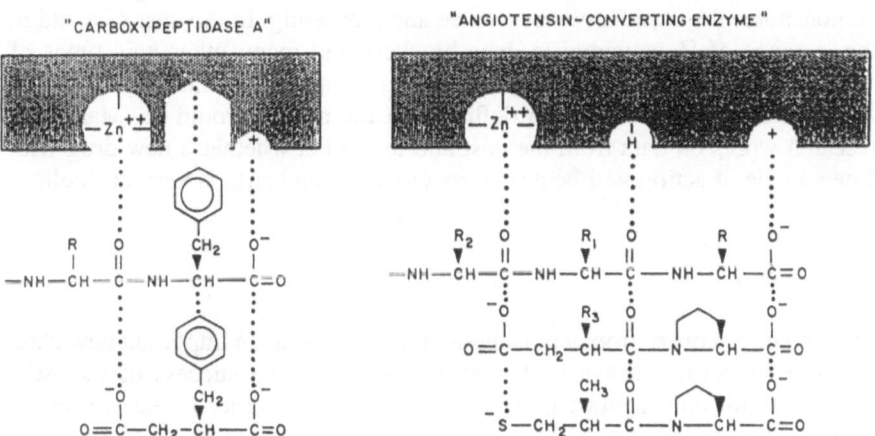

Figure 5   Schematic representation of the binding of substrates and inhibitors at the active site of pancreatic carboxypeptidase A, and at the hypothetical active site of angiotensin-converting enzyme (from [31] with permission).

Captopril was the final product of these studies in which only 60 compounds were synthesised and logically tested [31]. Interestingly, they had also set up a random screen for inhibitors of ACE and tested over 2000 compounds from the Squibb library. There were no positive leads.

As always, Merck was not far behind and they developed Enalapril and Lisinopril [31]. Here, then, was the birth of a new class of anti-hypertensive drugs, the ACE inhibitors. Between them, the first two alone (Captopril and Enalapril) sell billions of dollars each year. There are now at least ten other ACE inhibitors available in even more preparations and presentations. One of the shared side-effects of the ACE inhibitors has been the propensity to cause a cough and this has been ascribed to the inhibition of the breakdown of bradykinin.

There are many interesting aspects of this scientific trail from a poisonous snake venom to ACE inhibitors as valuable therapeutic agents. Serendipity, chance and coincidence all played a part. In the first place, Sergio Ferreira wanted to go to Oxford for his post-doc studies to work with Bill Paton. However, his wife wanted to take a PhD at the London School of Economics, which was just round the corner from my laboratories in the Royal College of Surgeons and so he came to work with me. Had he gone to Bill Paton, Captopril may not exist.

The bioassay and the blood-bathed organ technique were very powerful tools in the mid-1960s and 1970s for making important new discoveries. Without them, we would not have discovered how aspirin works [2], the metabolic functions of the pulmonary circulation [7], the conversion of angiotensin-I to II in the lungs [8–10], prostacyclin [32], and Salvador Moncada would not have discovered the identity of endothelium derived relaxing factor (EDRF) as nitric oxide [33].

This story, along with many others involving new block-busting drugs also demonstrates the clash between science and marketing. In this instance and in the instance of H_2 antagonists, beta-blockers and many other new types of drugs, the marketing arm of the company gave the new scientific concepts no support because they could not define what the market would be. Marketing research works on data from the past and to predict whether a new drug with a new mode of action will be a success was then, and still, is very difficult.

Conclusions

The trail of discovery from a poisonous snake venom to an important new class of anti-hypertensive drugs is described. Indirectly, the success of the ACE inhibitors, not only against hypertension but also in other diseases such as heart failure has led to a further class of drugs, the angiotensin antagonists.

Note added in proof
Since this article was first written, Ferreira has published a contribution on the history of ACE inhibitors, which is not too different from this one [34].

References

1 Vane JR, Flower RJ, Botting RM (1990) History of aspirin and its mechanism of action. *Stroke* 21: 12–23

2 Vane JR (1971) Inhibition of prostaglandin synthesis as a mechanism of action for aspirin-like drugs. *Nature New Biol* 231: 232–235

3 Vane JR, Bakhle YS, Botting RM (1998) Cyclooxygenases 1 and 2. *Annu Rev Pharmacol Toxicol* 38: 97–120

4 Tiegerstedt R, Bergman P G (1898) Niere und Kreislauf. *Skand Arch Physiol* 8: 223–271

5 Skeggs LTKahn JR, Shumway NP (1956) The preparation and function of the hypertensin-converting enzyme. *J Exp Med* 103: 295–299

6 Vane JR (1964) The use of isolated organs for detecting active substances in the circulating blood. *Brit J Pharmacol* 23: 360–373

7 Vane JR (1969) The release and fate of vaso-active hormones in the circulation. *Brit J Pharmacol* 35: 209–242

8 Ng KKF, Vane JR (1967) Conversion of angiotensin I to angiotensin II. *Nature* 216: 762–766

9 Bakhle YS, Reynard AM, Vane JR (1969) Metabolism of the Angiotensins in isolated perfused tissues. *Nature* 222: 956–959

10 Ng KKF, Vane JR (1968) Fate of angiotensin I in the circulation. *Nature* 218: 144–150

11 Yang HYT, Erdos EG, Levin Y (1971) Characterisation of a dipeptide hydrolase (kininase II: angiotensin converting enzyme). *J Pharmacol Exp Ther* 177: 291–298

12 Ryan JW, Ryan US, Schultz DR, Whitaker C, Chung A (1975) Subcellular localization of pulmonary angiotensin-converting enzyme (kininase II). *Biochem J* 146: 497–499

13 Ryan US (1986) Metabolic activity of endothelium: modulations of structure and function. *Annu Rev Physiol* 48: 263–277

14 Vane JR (1994) The Croonian Lecture, 1993. The endothelium: maestro of the blood circulation. *Phil Trans R Soc Lond* 343: 225–246

15 Regoli D, Vane JR (1966) The continuous estimation of angiotensin formed in the circulation of the dog. *J Physiol* 183: 513–531

16 Hodge RL, Lowe RD, Vane JR (1966) The effects of alteration of blood-volume on the concentration of circulating angiotensin In anaesthetized dogs. *J Physiol* 185: 613–626

17. Increased angiotensin formation in response to carotid occlusion in the dog. *Nature* 211: 491–493

18 Ferreira SH (1965) A bradykinin-potentiating factor (BPF) present in the venom of *Bothrops jararaca. Brit J Pharmacol* 24: 163–169

19 Ferreira SH, Vane JR (1967) The detection and estimation of bradykinin in the circulating blood. *Brit J Pharmacol* 29: 367–377

20 Ferreira SH, Vane JR (1967) The disappearance of bradykinin and eledoisin in the circulation and vascular beds of the cat. *Brit J Pharmacol* 30: 417–424

21 Ferreira SH, Vane JR (1967) Half-lives of peptides and amines in the circulation. *Nature* 215: 1237–1240

22 Bakhle YS (1968) Conversion of angiotensin I to angiotensin II by cell-free extracts of dog lung. *Nature* 220: 919–921

23 Aiken JW, Vane JR (1970) The renin-angiotensin system: inhibition of converting enzyme in isolated tissues. *Nature* 228: 30–34

24 Greene LJ, Camargo AC, Krieger EM, Stewart JM, Ferreira SH (1972) Inhibition of the conversion of angiotensin I to II and potentiation of bradykinin by small peptides present in *Bothrops jararaca* venom. *Circ Res* 30: 62–71

25 Ferreira SH, Bartelt DC, Greene LJ (1970) Isolation of bradykinin-potentiating peptides from *Bothrops jararaca* venom. *Biochemistry* 9: 2583–2593

26 Ondetti MA, Williams NJ, Sabo EF, Pluscec J, Weaver ER, Kocy O (1971) Angiotensin-converting enzyme inhibitors from the venom of *Bothrops jararaca:* Isolation, elucidation of structure, and synthesis. *Biochemistry* 10: 4033–4039

27 Collier JG, Robinson BF, Vane JR (1973) Reduction of the pressor effects of angiotensin In man by a synthetic nonapeptide (BPP$_{9a}$ or SQ 20,881) which inhibits converting enzyme. *Lancet* I: 72–74

28 Gavras H, Brunner HR, Laragh JH, Sealey JE, Gavras I, Vukovitch RA (1974) An angiotensin converting-enzyme inhibitor to identify and treat vasoconstrictor and volume factors in hypertensive patients. *N Engl J Med* 291: 817–821

29 Johnson JG, Black WD, Vukovitch RA, Hatch FEJr Friedman BI, Blackwell CF, Shenouda AN, Share L, Shade RE, Acchiardo SR et al (1974) Treatment of patients with severe hypertension by inhibition of converting enzyme. *Clin Sci Mol Med* 48: 53s–56s

30 Ondetti MA, Cushman DW (1984) Angiotensin-converting enzyme inhibition: Biochemical properties and biological actions. *CRC Crit Rev Biochem* 16: 381–411

31 Cushman DW, Ondetti MA (1991) History of the design of captopril and related inhibitors of angiotensin converting enzyme. *Hypertension* 17: 589–592

32 Moncada S, Vane JR (1979) Prostacyclin in perspective. *In*: JR Vane, S Bergstrom (eds): *Prostacyclin*. Raven Press, New York, 5–16

33 Palmer MJ, Ferrige AG, Moncada S (1987) Nitric oxide accounts for the biological activity of endothelium-derived relaxing factor. *Nature* 327: 524–526

34 Ferreira SH (2000) Angiotensin Converting enzyme: History and Relevance. *Semin Perinatol* 24: 7–10

ACE Inhibitors
ed. by P. D'Orléans-Juste and G.E. Plante
© 2001 Birkhäuser Verlag/Switzerland

Genetics of the renin-angiotensin-aldosterone system and risk of arterial disease

Malika Lajemi and Athanase Benetos

Unité INSERM 337, Institut des cordeliers, 15 rue de l'ecole de médecine, F-75006-Paris, France

Introduction

The activity of the renin-angiotensin-aldosterone (RAA) system is thought to play a significant role in the development of cardiovascular atherosclerotic and hypertensive disease. The RAA system plays an important role in the regulation of blood pressure, cardiac and arterial structure [1] and salt and water homeostasis. Also, this system is well-known to be involved in the control of blood pressure and the pathogenesis of several forms of experimental and human hypertension. Angiotensinogen is cleaved by renin to produce the inactive peptide angiotensin I [2]. The ACE then converts angiotensin I (Ang I) to angiotensin II (Ang II), the latter peptide has various effects including vasoconstriction, aldosterone production, and enhanced noradrenalin release from sympathetic nerve endings. Ang II has also hypertrophic, and possibly hyperplastic, effects on vascular smooth muscle cells and cardiomyocytes [3], and increases extracellular collagen matrix synthesis.

Two subtypes of angiotensin II receptors, angiotensin II type 1 receptor (AT1) and angiotensin II type 2 receptor (AT2), have been cloned and characterised [4–6]. Gene targeting approaches have suggested that both genes are involved in blood pressure regulation and modulation of the effect of angiotensin II in different manners [7–9]. The AT1 receptor is the primary receptor that mediates the vasoconstrictor and growth-promoting effects of angiotensin II in humans [10]. Angiotensin II-induced stimulation of AT1 receptors has on one hand direct effects on vascular smooth muscle cell contractility and synthetic activity, and the other hand stimulates the synthesis of aldosterone, the primary human mineralocorticoid, which acts on the distal nephron to regulate sodium resorption, potassium excretion, and intravascular volume. Activation of AT1 receptors stimulates the activity of aldosterone synthase (CYP11B2). Experimental studies have shown that aldosterone is a major stimulator of cardiac and vascular collagen synthesis [11]. Furthermore, the presence of aldosterone receptors in large arteries, especially in the aorta [12], and the discovery of endogenous vascular synthesis of aldosterone [13] suggest that this hormone plays a significant role in regulating the structure of large arteries.

A genetic epidemiological approach is useful to elucidate the genes responsible for hypertension. DNA libraries for the study of hypertension have been set up, and many informative genetic markers distributed along the genome have been identified. Most studies to date have relied on a case-control analysis to test an excess of molecular variants from the RAA system among hypertensive cases compared with normotensive controls. Genetic analyses of components of this system have succeeded in showing the importance of some proteins, such as angiotensin-converting enzyme (ACE) and angiotensinogen (AGT), in the pathogenesis of cardiovascular disease. Several diallelic polymorphisms have been detected in the coding and 3' untranslated regions of the angiotensin II type 1 receptor [14]. None of them is functionally relevant, but some associations with cardiovascular phenotypes have also been reported for one variant, an adenine to cytosine nucleotide transversion at the 1166 position [A^{1166}/C] located at the 5' end of the 3' untranslated region of the human AT1 gene [4]. More recently, a polymorphism in the regulatory region of the aldosterone synthase (CYP11B2) at the −344 position [T^{-344}C] has been examined and results suggest an involvement in the regulation of blood pressure and cardiovascular alterations.

Hypertension

Blood pressure is controlled by a variety of mechanisms that involve several genetic loci and environmental factors. However, little is known about the genes actually involved in human hypertension, about their respective importance in determining blood pressure, and about their interaction with other genes and environmental components. A number of epidemiological studies have shown that individual blood pressures result from both genetic predisposition and environmental factors. The heritable component of blood pressure has been documented in familial and twin studies. The evidence suggests that approximately 30% of the variance of blood pressure is attributable to genetic heritability and 50% to environmental influences [15].

Angiotensin-converting enzyme (ACE)

Since the identification of an insertion/deletion polymorphism in the ACE gene, numerous studies have evaluated the potential risk of the DD genotype in cardiovascular disease and hypertension. At the present time, an important part of these results are discrepant and could be explained by differences in the ethnical origin which affect the allele frequency, gender, body mass index, the degree of hypertension and, finally, environmental risk factors.

Although the ACE plays an important role in blood pressure regulation, no relationship between the insertion/deletion [I/D] polymorphism of the ACE gene and essential hypertension has been reported in many studies including European [16–18] and Japanese populations [19–21].

Other studies also showed a positive association between the D allele and high blood pressure in several populations (black American, white American, Japanese etc) [20, 22]. In a large, population-based sample, O'Donnell et al. [23] and Fornage et al. [24] revealed, in men but not in women, an association and genetic linkage of the ACE locus with hypertension and with diastolic blood pressure. However, more recently, Sugiyama et al. [21] did not observe such a sex-specific association. Nakano et al. [25] suggested that the ACE gene may participate in the regulation of blood pressure only in subjects with severe or resistant hypertension. In this study, the authors did not observe differences in age, blood pressure, or resting plasma renin activity (PRA) among ACE [I/D] genotypes. On the contrary, they reported an earlier onset of hypertension in subjects with the [DD] genotype.

Celantano et al. [26] show that after adjustment for other cardiovascular risk factors, such as smoking, hypercholesterolaemia, diabetes or genetic predisposition to hypertension, a linkage between the ACE [I/D] genotype and hypertension was observed. Subjects with a non-DD genotype expressed the lowest value of systolic and pulse blood pressures [26] and normotensive subjects with a familial history of hypertension and [DD] genotype expressed higher 24-hour systolic BP than subjects with [II] genotype [27]. Nevertheless, whatever the results of genotype-hypertension association, the ACE [I/D] polymorphism clearly affects the protein level. Indeed, plasma and tissue ACE concentrations have been found to correlate with the deletion (D) allele of the [I/D] polymorphism. Thus, the genetic effect accounts for 47% of the total variance of plasma ACE [28]. A similar observation was made in plasma ACE activity [29]. ACE plasma levels in patients with the [DD] genotype were 2-fold higher than in patients with the [II] genotype [30, 31]. As for plasma levels, ACE enzymatic activity is also higher in the presence of the ACE gene deletion polymorphism [28, 32–34] even in patients with coronary artery disease [31, 33, 35].

Angiotensinogen gene (AGT)

As for the ACE, the gene encoding for the angiotensinogen has been widely studied as a candidate gene for hypertension. The involvement of two frequent variants of the angiotensinogen gene, $[T^{174}M]$ (Thr–Met at amino acid position 174) and $[M^{235}T]$ (Met–Thr at amino acid position 235) located on exon 2, in human essential hypertension has been suggested in various populations and ethnic groups such as in white Europeans [36–38] and Japanese [39]. $[M^{235}T]$ is the genetic polymorphism the most studied with the ACE gene. Jeunemaitre et al. found the $[M^{235}T]$ variant of the AGT gene more frequently in hypertensive probands, especially in the more severe index cases, than in normotensive controls [36]. These findings were not replicated in other studies in Caucasians [17, 40, 41], African-Americans [42] and Chinese [43, 44]. Ethnic differences, affecting genotype and allele frequencies, probably explain an important part of the discrepant results. In this context, Ishigami et al. [19] showed that the allele frequency of $[M^{235}T]$, as with ACE [I/D], was different in the Japanese population than in the European-origin populations. Nevertheless, in a recent study, Vasku et al. [45] have compared a double homozygote combination of ACE gene and $[M^{235}T]$. A clear association between the [DDMM] genotype and essential hypertension was shown. On the contrary, no association of single gene allelic variants with essential hypertension was found for ACE [I/D] or $[M^{235}T]$ polymorphisms. Thus, the interaction of the ACE [I/D] and $[M^{235}T]$ AGT polymorphic alleles can contribute to essential hypertension, despite the absence of single gene association with the condition.

Interestingly, the $[M^{235}T]$ variant is potentially responsible for increased production of angiotensin II with a 10% and 20% increase in heterozygotes [MT] and homozygotes [TT], respectively, compared with wild-type homozygotes [MM] [36, 46]. Finally, plasma angiotensinogen level positively correlated with blood pressure (BP) in subjects with a positive family history of hypertension [47].

This variant seems also to be associated with the plasma concentration of other proteins from the RAA system. In a population survey in southern Germany, Danser et al. [48] revealed that the $M^{235}T$ allele of the angiotensinogen gene was related to lower plasma prorenin and renin levels, but not to plasma ACE and aldosterone, after adjustment for sex, age and blood pressure. In healthy normotensive subjects, angiotensinogen also significantly correlated with both body mass index (BMI) and plasma leptin. More precisely, circulating angiotensinogen levels seem to be associated with adipose mass in young normotensive, non-obese men who are genetically predisposed to the development of hypertension. Indeed, the abundant expression of angiotensinogen in human adipose tissue derived from omental and subcutaneous fat depots has been recently reported [36, 49]. These finding may point to a mechanism that counteracts the genetic elevation of angiotensinogen plasma levels, and thus the plasmatic angiotensin II-generating pathway, in subjects carrying the angiotensinogen $M^{235}T$ allele [48]. In other words, relationships exist between the angiotensinogen genotype, the intermediate phenotype (i.e., plasma angiotensinogen elevation), and the distal phenomenon (i.e., blood pressure elevation).

Angiotensin II type 1 receptor (AT1 R)

The AT1 $A^{1166}C$ variant was not shown to be associated with hypertension [50–52], except for one study [14]. In the latter study, the allelic frequency of $A^{1166}C$ was significantly increased in hypertensive subjects with a positive family history of hypertension or in patients with severe hypertension compared with normotensive control subjects. Furthermore, it has been recently reported that a [A^{1166}C] polymorphism of the AT1 gene occurs more frequently in resistant hypertensives taking two or more antihypertensive drugs [53]. In hypertensives, higher values of systolic blood pressure were associated with the C allele of the AT1 gene and only in older and overweight patients [53]. An association between the presence of the C allele and higher values of diastolic blood pressure was also present in overweight patients [53]. Such results suggest that in resistant hypertensive subjects the AT1 [A^{1166}C] polymorphism is potentially involved in the regulation of blood pressure and may amplify the effects of age and BMI on resistant essential hypertension.

A recent study aimed to determine whether Ang II AT1 receptors were influenced by the AT1 [A^{1166}C] genotype [54]. B(max) and K(D) values of the Ang II binding sites on platelets were calculated in 114 normotensive and hypertensive subjects to examine a possible relationship between these parameters and the AT1 [A^{1166}C] genotype. This study did not find any association between the AT1 [A^{1166}C] polymorphism and the AT1 receptor function.

Aldosterone synthase (CYP11B2)

Among genes coding for the RAA system, the CYP11B2 gene could play an important role in the development of hypertension and blood pressure regulation but, at the present time, very few studies have been reported and results are inconclusive. Several frequent polymorphisms have recently been described in the transcriptional regulatory region of the CYP11B2 gene, and particularly a [T^{-344}C] transversion.

As in Chilean patients [55], Takami et al. [56] described more recently that in Japanese hypertensive subjects, the [TC + CC] genotype was significantly associated with a higher aldosterone to plasma renin activity ratio (ALD/PRA). A high ratio of involved aldosterone to plasma renin activity recovers people with low renin hypertension. Pojoga et al. [57] also observed higher levels of aldosterone and lower levels of renin in the [CC] subjects compared to the [TT] genotype. The genotype [T^{-344}C] of CYP11B2 significantly associated with hypertension in the Japanese study. Also, the frequency of nondippers between the daytime and the nighttime was significantly higher in subjects with the [TC + CC] genotype than in subjects with the [TT] genotype. Other studies did not observe any association between this genotype and BP levels [57].

Left ventricular hypertrophy (LVH)

ACE I/D

The ACE [DD] genotype has been reported in clinical studies to be associated with left ventricular hypertrophy [26, 49, 58, 59]. However, the precise mechanism of this association remains unknown and some confounding factors might also affect the association. Results show first that the ACE genotype significantly and independently influences LVH and microalbuminuria [60] in normotensive subjects but not in hypertensive subjects [49, 61]. Studies revealed precisely that patients with [DD] and [ID] genotypes showed increased left ventricular mass compared with [II] patients [25, 60]. Nevertheless, other [62–65] studies, amongst which a large study based on the Framinghan study [66], found no evidence of an association between the ACE polymorphism and echocardiographically-determined left ventricular mass or electric LVH. In previously untreated hypertensive subjects, no evidence suggests that the deletion polymorphism of the ACE genotype is important in the development of LVH [63].

According to some [67–69], but not all [70, 71], studies the frequency of the D allele is also higher in patients with hypertrophic cardiomyopathy (HCM). The extent of hypertrophy in these subjects was influenced by the ACE [I/D] polymorphism [68, 70, 71] suggesting that the RAA system may modify the phenotypic expression of hypertrophy in HCM.

AGT

Two recent studies determined the relationship of the [$M^{235}T$] polymorphism of the AGT gene with left ventricular mass (LVM). In 175 Chinese patients with hypertension, Jeng et al. demonstrated that patients with the [TT] genotype were found to have a significantly greater LVM index than those with the [MM] and [MT] genotypes [72]. In a similar fashion, the angiotensinogen gene [$M^{235}T$] polymorphism is associated with the variability in left ventricular hypertrophy induced by endurance training, with athletes homozygous for the T allele having the largest hearts [73]. Thus, the [TT] genotype of the AGT gene could be considered as a risk factor for the development of cardiac hypertrophy. However, Kauma et al. [74] and Fernandez-Llama et al. [41] did not observe such a relationship in a middle-aged population-based cohort of hypertensives and control subjects. In fact, no differences in the adjusted left ventricular mass values in the [$M^{235}T$] AGT genotypes were seen among either the hypertensive or the control subjects [41, 74], or in the subgroups of physically active subjects [74]. Also, no association with the [$T^{174}M$] variant of the AGT was observed either with essential hypertension or with target organ damage such as left ventricular hypertrophy in a Spanish sample [41].

AT1 $A^{1166}C$

The angiotensin II AT1 $A^{1166}C$ allele may also be a candidate to affect left ventricular mass in Japanese normotensive subjects [52] and hypertensive subjects

[60]. Combined with other factors, it might contribute genetically to the increase in left ventricular mass in hypertensive and (HCM) patients. Nevertheless, patients with hypertensive LVH showed a higher $A^{1166}C$ allele frequency of AT1 compared to patients with HCM. In this context, Pontremoli et al. [60] have shown that patients with [DD] and [ID] genotypes expressed higher levels of the [A/C] $AT1^{1166}$ polymorphism and together increased left ventricular mass index compared with [II] patients. Carriers of both AT1 ^{1166}C and ACE [I/D] D alleles had a four-fold increase in the odds ratio for family history of HCM without manifesting the disease.

CYP11B2

The $T^{-344}C$ gene polymorphism of CYP11B2 has also been recently reported to be associated with left ventricular mass in young Finnish adults free of clinical heart disease [75] or in Japanese [56]. Echocardiographic assessment in hypertensive Japanese has revealed that the ratio of left ventricular end-diastolic dimension to height tended to be higher in subjects with the CYP11B2 [TC + CC] genotype than in subjects with the [TT] genotype [56].

Coronary artery disease (CAD)

Myocardial infarction (MI)

Coronary artery disease (CAD) is a polygenic and polyfactorial disease whose phenotypic manifestation depends on the interaction of a number of environmental factors. The first study to address the ACE DD type as a potential risk factor for MI was that of Cambien et al. in 1992 [31] who found a significant association particularly for individuals at low risk according to classical criteria. In several studies the ACE [I/D] gene polymorphism has been clearly demonstrated to be associated with myocardial infarction [31, 76]. Gene variants in the AT1 receptor gene $[A^{1166}C]$ have been found to interact with the ACE gene to increase the risk of MI [30]. Actually, the association between the ACE [DD] genotype and MI seemed to be restricted to a subset of individuals who carried the AT1 $[^{1166}$ C] allele. Consequently, the odds ratio for MI associated with the ACE [DD] genotype was four-fold higher in AT1 [CC] homozygote subjects than in [AA] homozygotes [77, 78]. Otherwise, among patients defined as low risk by traditional risk factors such as serum apolipoprotein B and BMI, the interaction between ACE [I/D] and the AT1 polymorphism was shown to be stronger [30]. The presence of classical factors seems to mask the effect of the [DD] genotype on cardiovascular diseases, since only in low risk patients is the association between the ACE polymorphism and cardiovascular diseases manifested (Tab. 1).

Table 1. Renin-angiotensin-aldosterone system gene polymorphisms and coronary artery disease

Coronary artery disease (CAD)	Genetic polymorphisms				
	AGT				
	$T^{174}M$ [TT]	$M^{235}T$ [TT + MT]	ACE I/D [DD]	AT1R $A^{1166}C$ [AC + CC]	CYP11B2 $T^{-344}C$ [TT + TC]
Prevalence of CAD	Cong et al. (1998) [79]	Cong et al. (1998) [79] Ludwig et al. (1997) [85] Ishigami et al. (1995) [84]	Cong et al. (1998) [79] Sigusch et al. (1997) [80] Gardemann et al. (1998) [81] Ferrieres et al. (1998) [82]		
Extent of coronary artery lesions		Jeunemaitre et al. (1997) [87] Sigusch et al. (1997) [80]	Pfohl et al. (1998) [88] Jeunemaitre et al. (1997) [87] Sigusch et al. (1997) [80]	Nakauchi et al. (1996) [91]	
Vascular tone				Amant et al. (1997) [92] Henrion et al. (1998) [93]	
Aortic stiffness and hypertrophy		Arnett et al. (1998) [107] Castellano et al. (1995) [108]	Arnett et al. (1998) [107] Castellano et al. (1995) [108]	Benetos et al. (1996) [105, 106]	Pojoga et al. (1998) [57]
Left ventricular hypertrophy		[TT]: Jeng et al. (1999) [72] Karjalainen et al. (1999) [73]	[NT]: Ohishi et al. (1994) [61] Iwai et al. (1994) [58] Schunkert et al. (1994) [49] Nakano et al. (1998) [25] Pontromeli et al. (1996) [60] Celentano et al. (1998) [26] (1999) [59]	[NT]: Takami et al. (1998) [52] [HT]: Pontromeli et al. (1996) [60] Jeng et al. (1999) [72] Karjalainen et al. (1999) [73]	[HT]: Kupari et al. (1998) [75] Takami et al. (1999) [56]
Myocardial infarction			Cambien et al. (1992) [31] Tiret et al. (1998) [76] Osterop et al. (1998) [77] Ishanov et al. (1998) [78]		

Positive associations were indicated by one or several reference articles. Letters in brackets designate one or two genotypes together. NT: normotensive and HT: hypertensive.

Prevalence of coronary artery disease (CAD)

Indeed, a strong association between the frequency of the ACE [DD] genotype and CAD was found in Japanese [79] and Caucasians [80–83]. Also, according to some studies, a significant association between coronary atherosclerosis and the AGT [M^{235}T] variant of angiotensinogen was found, again in Japanese populations with coronary atherosclerosis [19, 79]. Together, ACE [DD] and AGT ^{235}T gene homozygotes have been reported to correlate with an increased prevalence of CAD [36, 84, 85]. Furthermore, the relationship between coronary artery disease and the AGT 174 codon polymorphism was analysed in Japanese subjects with CAD or healthy subjects [79]. The results showed that the frequency of [TT] homozygotes of AGT codon 174 was significantly higher in CAD patients compared to controls [79]. This finding suggested that the [TT] genotype of AGT codon 174 may be a risk factor for CAD in Japanese individuals with low BMI, lesser CAD risk factors, or ACE [II] genotype.

Conversely, neither the [DD] genotype of the ACE [ID] polymorphism, nor the ^{174}T and ^{235}T homozygotes of the AGT gene conferred significant risk factor for CAD in a Chinese study [86].

Extent of coronary artery stenosis

Several studies showed a significant correlation between both the AGT ^{235}T allele or the ACE [I/D] D allele and the extent of the coronary lesions in patients with low or high cardiovascular risk (Tab. 1) [80, 87]. More precisely, Sigusch et al. [80] found that the [DD] genotype was significantly more common in patients having multi-vessel CAD as compared to controls and to patients with single vessel involvement (where the genotype distribution was not significantly different from controls). Pfohl et al. [88] have also shown that patients with CAD and the ACE [DD] genotype have a significantly higher incidence and greater extent of coronary lesion calcification. A few other studies showed that the D allele of ACE [ID] is not associated with the severity of coronary artery stenosis even in low risk patients [89, 90].

The AT1 C allele has been reported to be involved in the development of the coronary artery stenosis since the number of affected vessels was significantly greater in patients with the AT1 ^{1166}C allele than in those with the [AA] genotype [91].

Endothelial dysfunction, thrombosis

Endothelial cell dysfunction and coagulation activation play important roles in both the atherosclerotic process and the cardiovascular complications. Some observations support the attractive hypothesis that effects of the ACE [I/D] allele polymorphism on cardiovascular disease are mediated by altered expression of tissue and/or circulating ACE [34]. It should be a risk factor for the development of hypertensive cardiovascular disease associated with endothelial cell damage. Precisely, Singer et al. [34] have shown that Von Willebrand factor (vWF) and thrombomodulin were significantly higher in elderly hypertensive patients with the [DD] genotype than in those with the [ID] or [II] genotype. Positive correlation of systolic blood pressure with levels of both vWF and thrombomodulin were found predominantly in patients with the II genotype, but not with the DD genotype.

Vascular tone

Finally, the influence of the RAA genetic polymorphisms on coronary risk may be related, at least in part, to a deleterious effect on coronary vasomotion. Thus a recent study demonstrated that patients carrying the AT1 receptor [CC] genotype had significantly greater vasoconstriction in distal coronary vessels [92]. Similarly, an *in vitro* organ bath study on mammary artery from CAD patients provides evidence that the [A^{1166}C] genotype of the AT1 receptor is associated with a change in vascular reactivity [93].

   Taken together, these findings indicate that the gene polymorphisms of the renin-angiotensin-aldosterone system (ACE [I/D], AT1 A^{1166}C, AGT M^{235}T or T^{174}M, CYP11B2 T^{-344}C) could be involved in the development and the complications of ischemic heart disease through several mechanisms including severity of coronary atherosclerotic lesions, endothelial dysfunction, thrombosis and changes in vascular tone (Tab. 1). Genetic factors could also aggravate ischemic heart disease by altering the structure and the mechanical properties of aorta.

Aortic stiffness and hypertrophy

The two major causes of increased stiffness in the large arteries are age and high blood pressure. An increased mechanical stress caused by high blood pressure is a major determinant of arterial wall stiffness in hypertension [1, 94, 95]. As reported previously, aortic stiffness positively correlates with age and systolic blood pressure in both normotensive and hypertensive subjects [96, 97]. Increased stiffness is associated with several structural changes of the arterial wall, including arterial thickening and changes in extracellular matrix.

   In addition to age and high blood pressure, local hormonal factors may play a pressure-independent role on the arterial wall, mainly by modifying cell growth or synthesis of the extracellular matrix [98–102]. Among these factors angiotensin II might be of particular importance, since it induces hypertrophy of vascular smooth muscle cells in culture and increases collagen production by fibroblasts [100, 101]. *In vivo* administration of nonpressor doses of angiotensin II induces arterial thickening in rats [102], whereas in humans, higher levels of ACE have been observed in subjects with increased thickness of the carotid wall [103].

In clinical studies, the involvement of RAA gene polymorphisms on arterial stiffness and aortic distensibility were investigated in normotensive and hypertensive subjects [104–106]. We suggested that the AT1 gene is involved in the development of aortic stiffness in hypertensive patients, whereas these results were not observed in normotensive subjects (Tab. 1). The C allele frequency (25%) of AT1 was associated with a strong aortic stiffness after adjustment for age and blood pressure. Moreover, an interaction was found between AT1 genotype and the ratio of total to high-density lipoprotein cholesterol in terms of the development of aortic stiffness. Thus, a positive correlation was observed between the ratio of total to high-density lipoprotein cholesterol and pulse wave velocity (PWV) in [AC] and [CC] but not [AA] patients. The ACE [ID] polymorphism seems to play a less important role in determination of the arterial stiffness [106]. When compared to the homozygote [TT] subjects from the [T^{-344}C] polymorphism of CYP11B2, the C allele subjects expressed an elevated arterial stiffness.

With regard to the other gene polymorphisms from the RAA system, only a few studies have been reported. ACE [I/D] and AGT ^{235} T polymorphisms appeared associated with carotid intima-media thickness in a population-based sample of middle aged adults with no history of cardiovascular disease [107, 108]. Others studies did not confirm these observations [109].

Concluding remarks

In the last eight years a large number of clinical studies have attempted to assess the role of polymorphic variants of the RAA system on hypertension and cardiovascular disease and their complications. While many of these results suggest an important role for these genes in cardiovascular disease, especially the ACE [I/D] polymorphism, we cannot confirm that one or more of these genes are major contributors to cardiac disease.

Since essential hypertension and atherosclerosis are multifactorial and multigenic diseases, several genes could modulate the effects of environmental factors. The study of the role of genetic polymorphisms on the cardiovascular system should elucidate the interactions between several genes and environmental factors on precise cardiac and arterial phenotypes.

References

1 Dzau V, Safar M (1988) Large conduit arteries in hypertension: role of the renin-angiotensin system. *Circulation* 77: 947–953
2 Badenhop R, Wang X, Wilcken D (1996) Association between an angiotensinogen microsatellite marker in children and coronary events in their grandparents. *Circulation* 93: 2092–2096

3   Sadoshima J, Izumo S (1993) Molecular characterization of angiotensin II induced hypertrophy of
    cardiac myocytes and hyperplasia of cardiac fibroblast: critical role of AT1 receptor subtype. *Circ
    Res* 73: 413–423
4   Furuta H, Guo D, Inagami T (1992) Molecular cloning and sequencing of the gene encoding
    human angiotensin II type 1 receptor. *Biochem Biophys Res Commun* 183: 8–13
5   Guo D, Furuta H, Mizukoshi M, Inagami T (1994) The genomic organization of human
    angiotensin II type 1 receptor. *Biochem Biophys Res Commun* 200: 313–319
6   Koike G, Horiuchi M, Yamada T, Szpirer C, Jacob HJ, Dzau VJ (1994) Human type 2
    angiotensin II receptor gene: cloned, mapped to the X chromosome, and its mRNA is expressed
    in the human lung. *Biochem Biophys Res Commun* 203: 1842–1850
7   Ito M, Oliverio M, Mannon P, Best CF, Maeda N, Smithies O, Coffman TM (1995) Regulation of
    blood pressure by the type 1a angiotensin II receptor gene. *Proc Natl Acad Sci USA* 92:
    3521–3525
8   Ichiki T, Labosky P, Shiota C, Okuyama S, Imagawa Y, Fogo A, Niimura F, Ichikawa I, Hogan BL,
    Inagami T (1995) Effect on blood pressure and exploratory behaviour of mice lacking
    angiotensin II type-2 receptor. *Nature* 377: 748–750
9   Hein L, Barsh G, Pratt R, Dzau VJ, Kobilka BK (1995) Behavioural and cardiovascular effects of
    disrupting the angiotensin II type-2 receptor gene in mice. *Nature* 377: 744–747
10 Smith R, Timmermans P (1994) Human angiotensin receptor subtypes. *Curr Opin Nephrol
    Hypertension* 3: 112–122
11 Weber K, Brilla C (1991) Pathological hypertrophy and cardiac interstitium. *Circulation* 83:
    1849–1865
12 White P, Curnow K, Pascoe L (1994) Disorders of steroid 11 beta-hydroxylase isozymes.
    Endocrine Rev 15: 421–438
13 Takeda Y, Miyamori I, Yoneda T, Iki K, Hatakeyama H, Blair IA, Hsieh FY, Takeda R (1995)
    Production of aldosterone in isolated rat blood vessels. *Hypertension* 25: 170–173
14 Bonnardeaux A, Davies E, Jeunemaitre X, Féry I, Charru A, Clauser E, Tiret L, Cambien F, Corvol
    P, Soubrier F (1994) Angiotensin II type 1 receptor gene polymorphisms in human essential hyper-
    tension. *Hypertension* 24: 63–69
15 Ward R (ed.) (1990) *Familial aggregation and genetic epidemiology of blood pressure*. Raven
    Press, New York
16 Barley J, Blackwood A, Miller M, Markandu N, Carter N, Jeffery S, Cappuccio F, MacGregor G,
    Sagnella G (1996) Angiotensin converting enzyme gene I/D polymorphism, blood pressure and
    the renin-angiotensin system in caucasian and afro-carribbean peoples. *J Hum Hypertens* 10:
    31–35
17 Mondorf U, Russ A, Wiesemann A, Herrero M, Oremek G, Lenz T (1998) Contribution of
    angiotensin I converting enzyme gene polymorphism and angiotensinogen gene polymorphism to
    blood pressure regulation in essential hypertension. *Amer J Hypertens* 11: 174–183
18 Kario K, Matsuo T, Kobayashi H, Kanai N, Hoshide S, Mitsuhashi T, Ikeda U, Nishiuma S,
    Matsuo M, Shimada K (1998) Endothelial cell damage and angiotensin-converting enzyme inser-
    tion/deletion genotype in elderly hypertensive patients. *J Amer Coll Cardiol* 32: 444–450
19 Ishigami T, Iwamoto T, Tamura K, Yamaguchi S, Iwasawa K, Uchino K, Umemura S, Ishii M
    (1995) Angiotensin I converting enzyme (ACE) gene polymorphism and essential hypertension in
    japan. Ethnic difference of ACE genotype. *Amer J Hypertens* 8: 95–97
20 Wuyts B, Delanghe J, De Buyzere M (1997) Angiotensin I-converting enzyme insertion/deletion
    polymorphism: clinical implications. *Acta Clin Belg* 52: 338–349
21 Sugiyama T, Morita H, Kato N, Kurihara H, Yamori Y, Yazaki Y (1999) Lack of sex-specific
    effects on the association between angiotensin-converting enzyme gene polymorphism and hyper-
    tension in japanese. *Hypertens Res* 22: 55–59
22 Abbud Z, Wilson A, Cosgrove N, Kostis J (1998) Angiotensin-converting enzyme gene polymor-
    phism in systemic hypertension. *Amer J Cardiol* 81: 244–246
23 O'Donnell C, Lindpaintner K, Larson M, Rao V, Ordovas J, Schaefer E, Myers R, Levy D (1998)
    Evidence for association and genetic linkage of the angiotensin-converting enzyme locus with
    hypertension and blood pressure in men but not women in the framingham heart study. *Circulation*
    97: 1766–1772
24 Fornage M, Amos C, Kardia S, Sing C, Turner S, Boerwinkle E (1998) Variation in the region of
    the angiotensin-converting enzyme gene influences interindividual differences in blood pressure
    levels in young white males. *Circulation* 97: 1773–1779

25 Nakano Y, Oshima T, Hiraga H, Matsuura H, Kajiyama G, Kambe M (1998) DD genotype of the angiotensin I-converting enzyme gene is a risk factor for early onset of essential hypertension in japanese patients. *J Lab Clin Med* 131: 502–506

26 Celentano A, Mancini F, Crivaro M, Palmieri V, De Stefano V, Ferrara LA, Di Minno G, De Simone G (1998) Influence of cardiovascular risk factors on the relation between angiotensin converting enzyme-gene polymorphism and blood pressure in arterial hypertension. *J Hypertension* 16: 985–991

27 Chrostowska M, Narkiewicz K, Bigda J, Winnicki M, Pawlowski R, Rossi G, Krupa-Wojciechowska B (1998) Ambulatory systolic blood pressure is related to the deletion allele of the angiotensin I converting enzyme gene in young normotensives with parental history of hypertension. *Clin Exp Hypertension* 20: 283–294

28 Rigat B, Hubert C, Alhenc-Gelas F, Cambien F, Corvol P, Soubrier F (1990) An insertion/deletion polymorphism in the angiotensin I converting enzyme gene accounting for half the variance of serum enzyme levels. *J Clin Invest* 86: 1343–1346

29 Lee E (1994) Population genetics of the angiotensin-converting enzyme in Chinese. *Brit J Clin Pharmacol* 37: 212–214

30 Tiret L, Bonnardeaux A, Poirier O, Ricard S, Marques-Vidal P, Evans A, Arveiler D, Luc G, Kee F, Ducimetière P et al (1994) Synergistic effects of angiotensin-converting enzyme and angiotensin-II type 1 receptor gene polymorphisms on risk of myocardial infarction. *Lancet* 344: 910–913

31 Cambien F, Poirier O, Lecerf L, Evans A, Cambou J, Arveiler D, Luc G, Bard J, Bara L, Ricard S et al (1992) Deletion polymorphism in the gene for angiotensin-converting enzyme is a potent risk factor for myocardial. *Nature* 359: 641–644

32 Cambien F, Costerousse O, Tiret L, Poirier O, Lecerf L, Gonzales M, Evans A, Arveiler D, Cambou J, Luc G et al (1994) Plasma level and gene polymorphism of angiotensin-converting enzyme in relation to myocardial infarction. *Circulation* 90: 669–676

33 Nakai K, Itoh C, Miura Y, Hotta K, Musha T, Itoh T, Miyakawa T, Iwasaki R, Hiramori K (1994) Deletion polymorphism of the angiotensin I-converting enzyme gene associated with serum ACE concentration and increased risk for CAD in the japanese. *Circulation* 90: 2199–2202

34 Singer D, Missouris C, Jeffery S (1996) Angiotensin-converting enzyme gene polymorphism. What to do about all the confusion. *Circulation* 94: 236–239

35 Missouris C, Barley J, Jeffery S, Carter N, Singer D, Mac-Gregor G (1996) Genetic risk for renal artery stenosis: association with deletion polymorphism in angiotensin I-converting enzyme gene. *Kidney Int* 49: 534–537

36 Jeunemaitre X, Soubrier F, Kotelevtsev Y, Lifton R, Williams C, Charru A, Hunt S, Hopkins P, Williams R, Lalouel J, Corvol P (1992) Molecular basis of human hypertension: Role of angiotensinogen. *Cell* 71: 169–180

37 Caulfield M, Lavender P, Farrall M, Munroe P, Lawson M, Turner P, Clark A (1994) Linkage of the angiotensinogen gene to essential hypertension. *N Engl J Med* 330: 1629–1633

38 Tiret L, Ricard S, Poirier O, Arveiler D, Cambou J, Luc G, Evans A, Nicaud V, Cambien F (1995) Genetic variation at the angiotensinogen locus in relation to high blood pressure and myocardial infarction: the ECTIM study. *J Hypertension* 13: 311–317

39 Hata A, Namikawa C, Sasaki M, Sato K, Nakamura T, Tamura K, Lalouel JM (1994) Angiotensinogen as a risk factor for essential hypertension in Japan. *J Clin Invest* 93: 1285–1287

40 Bennett C, Schrader A, Morris B (1993) Cross-sectional analysis of Met235-Thr variant of angiotensinogen gene in severe, familial hypertension. *Biochem Biophys Res Commun* 197: 833–839

41 Fernandez-Llama P, Poch E, Oriola J, Botey A, Rivera F, Revert L (1998) Angiotensinogen gene M235T and T174M polymorphisms in essential hypertension. Relation with target organ damage. *Amer J Hypertens* 11: 439–444

42 Rotimi C, Cooper R, Ward R, Morrison L (1994) The role of the angiotensinogen gene in human hypertension: absence of an association among African Americans (abstract). *Genet Epidemiol* 11: 339

43 Niu T, Xu X, Rogus J, Zhou Y, Chen C, Yang J, Fang Z, Schmitz C, Zhao J, Rao V et al (1998) Angiotensinogen gene and hypertension in chinese. *J Clin Invest* 101: 188–194

44 Cheung B, Leung R, Shiu S, Tan K, Lau C, Kumana C (1998) M235T polymorphism of the angiotensinogen gene and hypertension in Chinese. *J Hypertension* 16: 1137–1140

45 Vasku A, Soucek M, Znojil V, Rihacek I, Tschoplova S, Strelcova L, Cidl K, Blazkova M, Hajek

D, Holla L et al (1998) Angiotensin I-converting enzyme and angiotensinogen gene interaction and prediction of essential hypertension. *Kidney Int* 53: 1479–1482

46 Jeunemaitre X, Charru A, Chatellier G, Dumont C, Sassano P, Soubrier F, Ménard J, Corvol P (1993) M235T variant of the human angiotensinogen gene in unselected hypertensive patients. *J Hypertension* 11 (suppl 5): S80–S81

47 Schorr U, Blaschke K, Turan S, Distler A, Sharma A (1998) Relationship between angiotensinogen, leptin and blood pressure levels in young normotensive men. *J Hypertension* 16: 1475–1480

48 Danser A, Derkx F, Hense H, Jeunemaitre X, Riegger G, Schunkert H (1998) Angiotensin (M235T) and angiotensin-converting enzyme (I/D) polymorphisms in association with plasma renin and prorenin levels. *J Hypertension* 16: 1879–1883

49 Schunkert H, Hense H, Holmer S, Stender M, Perz S, Keil U, Lorell B, Riegger G (1994) Association between a deletion polymorphism of the angiotensin-converting enzyme gene and left ventricular hypertrophy. *N Engl J Med* 30: 1634–1638

50 Castellano M, Muiesan M, Beschi M, Rizzoni D, Cinelli A, Salvetti M, Pasini G, Porteri E, Bettoni G, Zulli R et al (1996) Angiotensin II type 1 receptor A/C1166 polymorphism. Relationships with blood pressure and cardiovascular structure. *Hypertension* 28: 1076–1080

51 Schmidt S, Beige J, Walla-friedel M, Michel M, Sharma A, Ritz E (1997) A polymorphism in the gene for the angiotensin II type 1 receptor is not associated with hypertension. *J Hypertension* 15: 1385–1388

52 Takami S, Katsuya T, Rakugi H, Sato N, Nakata Y, Kamitani A, Miki T, Higaki J, Ogihara T (1998) Angiotensin II type 1 receptor gene polymorphism is associated with increase of left ventricular mass but not with hypertension. *Amer J Hypertens* 11: 316–321

53 Szombathy T, Szalai C, Katalin B, Palicz T, Romics L, Csaszar A (1998) Association of angiotensin II type 1 receptor polymorphism with resistant essential hypertension. *Clin Chim Acta* 269: 91–100

54 Paillard F, Chansel D, Brand E, Benetos A, Thomas F, Czekalski S, Ardaillou R, Soubrier F (1999) Genotype-phenotype relationships for the renin-angiotensin-aldosterone system in a normal population [In Process Citation]. *Hypertension* 34: 423–429

55 Fardella C, Rodriguez H, Montero J, Zhang G, Vignolo P, Rojas A, Villarroel L, Miller W (1996) Genetic variation in P450c11AS in chilean patients with low renin hypertension. *J Clin Endocrinol Metab* 81: 4347–4351

56 Tamaki S, Iwai N, Tsujita Y, Kinoshita M (1999) Genetic polymorphism of CYP11B2 gene and hypertension in japanese. *Hypertension* 33: 266–270

57 Pojoga L, Gautier S, Blanc H, Guyene TT, Poirier O, Cambien F, Benetos A (1998) Genetic determination of plasma aldosterone levels in essential hypertension. *Amer J Hypertens* 11: 856–860

58 Iwai N, Ohmichi N, Nakamura Y, Kinoshita M (1994) DD genotype of the angiotensin-converting enzyme gene is a risk factor for left ventricular hypertrophy. *Circulation* 90: 2622–2628

59 Celentano A, Mancini F, Crivaro M, Palmieri V, Ferrara L, De Stefano V, Di Minno G, De Simone G (1999) Cardiovascular risk factors, angiotensin-converting enzyme gene I/D polymorphism, and left ventricular mass in systemic hypertension. *Amer J Cardiol* 83: 1196–1200

60 Pontremoli R, Sofia A, Tirotta A, Ravera M, Nicolella C, Viazzi F, Bezante G, Borgia L, Bobola N, Ravazzolo R et al (1996) The deletion polymorphism of the angiotensin I-converting enzyme gene is associated with target organ damage in essential hypertension. *J Amer Soc Nephrol* 7: 2550–2558

61 Ohishi M, Rakugi H, Ogihara T (1994) Association between a deletion polymorphism of the angiotensin-converting enzyme and left ventricular hypertrophy. *N Engl J Med* 331: 1097–1098

62 West M, Summers K, Burstow D, Wong K, Huggard P (1994) Renin and angiotensin-converting enzyme genotypes in patients with essential hypertension and left ventricular hypertrophy. *Clin Exp Pharmacol Physiol* 21: 207–210

63 Mayet J, O'Kane K, Elton R, Johnstone H, Shahi M, Ozkor M, Stanton A, Poulter N, Sever P, Foale R et al (1997) Left ventricular hypertrophy, blood pressure and ACE genotype in untreated hypertension. *J Hum Hypertens* 11: 595–597

64 West M, Summers K, Wong K, Burstow D (1997) Renin-angiotensin system gene polymorphisms and left ventricular hypertrophy. The case against an association. *Adv Exp Med Biol* 432: 117–122

65 Hamon M, Amant C, Bauters C, Richard F, Helbecque N, McFadden E, Lablanche J, Bertrand M, Amouyel P (1997) Association of angiotensin converting enzyme and angiotensin II type 1 receptor genotypes with left ventricular function and mass in patients wwith angiographically normal coronary arteries. *Heart* 77: 502–505

66 Lindpaintner K, Lee M, Larson M, Rao V, Pfeffer M, Ordovas J, Schaefer E, Wilson A, Wilson P, Vasan R et al (1996) Absence for association or genetic linkage between the angiotensin-converting enzyme and left ventricular mass. *N Engl J Med* 334: 1023–1028

67 Pfeufer A, Osterziel K, Urara H, Borck G, Schuster H, Wienker TR, Luft F (1996) Angiotensin-converting enzyme and heart chymase gene polymorphisms in hypertrophic cardiomyopathy. *Amer J Cardiol* 78: 362–364

68 Yoneya K, Okamoto H, Machida M, Onozuka H, Noguchi M, Mikami T, Kawaguchi H, Murakami M, Uede T, Kitabatake A (1995) Angiotensin-converting enzyme gene polymorphism in japanese patients with hypertrophic cardiomyopathy. *Amer Heart J* 130: 1089–1093

69 Marian A, Yu Q, Workman R, Greve G, Roberts R (1993) Angiotensin-converting enzyme polymorphism in hypertrophic cardiomyopathy and sudden cardiac death. *Lancet* 342: 1085–1086

70 Tesson F, Dufour C, Moolman J, Carrier L, Al-Mahdawi S, Chojnowska L, Dubourg O, Soubrier F, Brink P, Komajda M et al (1997) The influence of the angiotensin I converting enzyme genotype in familial hypertrophic cardiomyopathy varies with the disease gene mutation. *J Mol Cell Cardiol* 29: 831–838

71 Lechin M, Quinones M, Omran A, Hill R, Yu Q, Rakowski H, Wigle D, Liew C, Sole M, Roberts R (1995) Angiotensin I converting enzymes genotypes and left ventricular hypertrophy in patients with hypertrophic cardiomyopathy. *Circulation* 92: 1808–1812

72 Jeng JR (1999) Left ventricular mass, carotid wall thickness, and angiotensinogen gene polymorphism in patients with hypertension. *Amer J Hypertens* 12: 443–450

73 Karjalainen J, Kujala UM, Stolt A, Mantysaari M, Viitasalo M, Kainulainen K, Kontula K (1999) Angiotensinogen gene M235T polymorphism predicts left ventricular hypertrophy in endurance athletes. *J Amer Coll Cardiol* 34: 494–499

74 Kauma H, Ikaheimo M, Savolainen MJ, Kiema TR, Rantala AO, Lilja M, Reunanen A, Kesaniemi YA (1998) Variants of renin-angiotensin system genes and echocardiographic left ventricular mass. *Eur Heart J* 19: 1109–1117

75 Kupari M, Hautanen A, Lankinen L, Koskinen P, Virolainen J, Nikkila H, White P (1998) Associations between human aldosterone synthase (CYP11B2) gene polymorphisms and left ventricular size, mass, and function. *Circulation* 97: 569–575

76 Tiret L, Blanc H, Ruidavets J, Arveiler D, Luc G, Jeunemaitre X, Tichet J, Mallet C, Poirier O, Plouin P et al (1998) Gene polymorphisms of the renin-angiotensin system in relation to hypertension and parental history of myocardial infarction and stroke: the PEGASE study. *J Hypertension* 16: 37–44

77 Osterop A, Kofflard MJM, Sandkuijl LA, Ten Cate FJ, Krams R, Schalekamp M, Danser A (1998) AT1 receptor A/C1166 polymorphism contributes to cardiac hypertrophy in subjects with hypertrophic cardiomyopathy. *Hypertension* 32: 825–830

78 Ishanov A, Okamoto H, Watanabe M, Yoneya K, Nakagawa I, Kumamoto H, Chiba S, Hata A, Kawaguchi H, Kitabatake A (1998) Angiotensin II type 1 receptor gene polymorphisms in patients with cardiac hypertrophy. *Jpn Heart J* 39: 87–96

79 Cong ND, Hamaguchi K, Saikawa T, Hara M, Sakata T (1998) A polymorphism of angiotensinogen gene codon 174 and coronary artery disease in Japanese subjects. *Amer J Med* 316: 339–344

80 Sigusch HH, Vogt S, Gruber U, Reinhardt D, Lang K, Surber R, Farker K, Muller S, Hoffmann A (1997) Angiotensin-I-converting enzyme DD genotype is a risk factor of coronary artery disease. *Scand J Clin Lab Invest* 57: 127–132

81 Gardemann A, Fink M, Stricker J, Nguyen Q, Humme J, Katz N, Tillmanns H, Hehrlein F, Rau M, Haberbosch W (1998) ACE I/D gene polymorphism: presence of the ACE D allele increases the risk of coronary artery disease in younger individuals. *Arteriosclerosis* 139: 153–159

82 Ferrieres J, Ruidavets J, Fauvel J, Perret B, Taraszzkiewicz D, Fourcade J, Nieto M, Chap H, Puel J (1999) Angiotensin I-converting enzyme gene polymorphism in a low-risk European population for coronary artery disease. *Arteriosclerosis* 142: 211–216

83 Alvarez R, Reguero JR, Batalla A, Iglesias-Cubero G, Cortina A, Alvarez V, Coto E (1998) Angiotensin-converting enzyme and angiotensin II receptor 1 polymorphisms: association with early coronary disease. *Cardiovasc Res* 40: 375–379

84 Ishigami T, Umemura S, Iwamoto T, Tamura K, Hibi K, Yamaguchi S, Nyuui N, Kimura K, Miyazaki N, Ishii M (1995) Molecular variant of angiotensinogen gene is associated with coronary atherosclerosis. *Circulation* 91: 951–954

85 Ludwig E, Borecki I, Ellison R, Folsom A, Heiss G, Higgins M, Lalouel J, Province M, Rao D (1997) Associations between candidate loci angiotensin-converting enzyme and angiotensinogen

with coronary heart disease and myocardial infarction: the NHLBI family heart study. *Ann Epidemiol* 7: 3–12

86 Ko YL, Ko YS, Wang SM, Chu PH, Teng MS, Cheng NJ, Chen WJ, Hsu TS, Kuo CT, Chiang CW et al (1997) Angiotensinogen and angiotensin-I converting enzyme gene polymorphisms and the risk of coronary artery disease in Chinese. *Hum Genet* 100: 210–214

87 Jeunemaitre X, Ledru F, Battaglia S, Guillanneuf MT, Courbon D, Dumont C, Darmon O, Guize L, Guermonprez JL, Diebold B et al (1997) Genetic polymorphisms of the renin-angiotensin system and angiographic extent and severity of coronary artery disease: the CORGENE study. *Hum Genet* 99: 66–73

88 Pfohl M, Athanasiadis A, Koch M, Clemens P, Benda N, Häring H, Karsch K (1998) Insertion/deletion polymorphism of the angiotensin I-converting enzyme gene is associated with coronary plaque calcification as assessed by intravascular ultrasound. *J Amer Coll Cardiol* 31: 987–991

89 Ludwig E, Corneli P, Anderson J, Marshall H, Lalouel J, Ward R (1995) Angiotensin-converting enzyme gene polymorphism is associated with myocardial infarction but not with development of coronary stenosis. *Circulation* 91: 2120–2124

90 Arca M, Pannitteri G, Campagna F, Candeloro A, Montali A, Cantini R, Seccareccia F, Campa PP, Marino B, Ricci G (1998) Angiotensin-converting enzyme gene polymorphism is not associated with coronary atherosclerosis and myocardial infarction in a sample of Italian patients. *Eur J Clin Invest* 28: 485–490

91 Nakauchi Y, Suehiro T, Yamamoto M, Yasuoka N, Arii K, Kumon Y, Hamashige N, Hashimoto K (1996) Significance of angiotensin I-converting enzyme and angiotensin II type 1 receptor gene polymorphisms as risk factors for coronary heart disease. *Atherosclerosis* 125: 161–169

92 Amant C, Hamon M, Bauters C, Richard F, Helbecque N, McFadden EP, Escudero X, Lablanche JM, Amouyel P, Bertrand ME (1997) The angiotensin II type 1 receptor gene polymorphism is associated with coronary artery vasoconstriction. *J Amer Coll Cardiol* 29: 486–490

93 Henrion D, Benessiano J, Philip I, Plantefève G, Chatel D, Hwas U, Desmont J, Durand G, Amouyel P, Lévy B (1998) Angiotensin II type 1 receptor gene polymorphism is associated with an increased vascular reactivity in the human mammary artery *in vitro*. *J Vasc Res* 35: 356–362

94 Safar M (1988) Therapeutic trials and large arteries in hypertension. *Amer Heart J* 115: 702–710

95 Nichols W, O'rourke M (eds) (1990) *McDonald's Blood Flow in Arteries: Theoretical, Experimental and Clinical Principles*. E Arnold, London, UK, 77–142, 216–269, 283–359, 398–437

96 Smulyan H, Csermely T, Mookherjee S, Warner R (1983) Effect of age on arterial distensibility in asymptomatic humans. *Arteriosclerosis* 3: 199–205

97 Asmar R, Benetos A, London G, Hugue C, Weiss Y, Topouchian J, Laloux B, Safar M (1995) Aortic distensibility in normotensive, untreated and treated hypertensive patients. *Blood Press* 4: 48–54

98 Dostal D, Baker K (1992) Angiotensin II stimulation of left ventricular hypertrophy in adult rat heart: mediation by the AT1 receptor. *Amer J Hypertens* 5: 276–280

99 Morishita R, Gibbons G, Ellison K, Lee W, Zhang L, Yu H, Kaneda Y, Ogihara T, Dzau V (1994) Evidence for direct local effect of angiotensin In vascular hypertrophy: *in vivo* gene transfer of angiotensin converting enzyme. *J Clin Invest* 94: 978–984

100 Bunkenburg B, Van Amelsvoort T, Rogg H, Wood J (1992) Receptor-mediated effects of angiotensin II on growth of vascular smooth muscle cells from spontaneously hypertensive rats. *Hypertension* 20: 746–754

101 Naftilan A, Pratt R, Dzau V (1989) Induction of c-fos, c-myc and PDGF A chain gene expression by angiotensin II in cultured rat vascular smooth muscle cells. *J Clin Invest* 83: 1419–1424

102 Griffin S, Brown W, Macpherson F, Macgrath J, Wilson V, Korsgaard N, Mulvany M, Lever A (1991) Angiotensin II causes vascular hypertrophy in part by a nonpressor mechanism. *Hypertension* 17: 626–635

103 Bonithon-Kopp C, Ducimetière P, Touboul P, Fève J, Billaud E, Courbon D, Héraud V (1994) Plasma angiotensin-converting enzyme activity and carotid wall thickening. *Circulation* 89: 952–954

104 Benetos A, Topouchian J, Ricard S, Gautier S, Bonnardeaux A, Asmar R, Poirier O, Soubrier F, Safar M, Cambien F (1995) Influence of angiotensin II type 1 receptor polymorphism on aortic stiffness in never-treated hypertensive patients. *Hypertension* 26: 44–47

105 Benetos A, Cambien F, Gautier S, Ricard S, Safar M, Laurent S, Lacolley P, Poirier O,

Topouchian J, Asmar R (1996) Influence of the angiotensin II type 1 receptor gene polymorphism on the effects of perindopril and nitrendipine on arterial stiffness in hypertensive individuals. *Hypertension* 28: 1081–1084

106 Benetos A, Gautier S, Ricard S, Topouchian J, Asmar R, Poirier O, Larosa E, Guize L, Safar M, Soubrier F et al (1996) Influence of angiotensin-converting enzyme and angiotensin II type 1 receptor gene polymorphisms on aortic stiffness in normotensive and hypertensive patients. *Circulation* 94: 698–703

107 Arnett DK, Borecki IB, Ludwig EH, Pankow JS, Myers R, Evans G, Folsom AR, Heiss G, Higgins M (1998) Angiotensinogen and angiotensin converting enzyme genotypes and carotid atherosclerosis: the atherosclerosis risk in communities and the NHLBI family heart studies. *Atherosclerosis* 138: 111–116

108 Castellano M, Muiesan M, Rizzoni D, Beschi M, Pasini G, Cinelli A, Salvetti M, Porteri E, Bettoni G, Kreutz R et al (1995) Angiotensin-converting enzyme I/D polymorphism and arterial wall thickness in a general population. The vobarno study. *Circulation* 91: 2721–2724

109 Barley J, Markus H, Brown M, Carter N (1995) Lack of association between angiotensinogen polymorphism (M235T) and cerebrovascular disease and carotid atheroma. *J Hum Hypertens* 9: 681–683

ACE Inhibitors
ed. by P. D'Orléans-Juste and G.E. Plante
© 2001 Birkhäuser Verlag/Switzerland

Crosstalk between ACE inhibitors, B_2 kinin receptor and nitric oxide in endothelial cells

Paulus Wohlfart, Gabriele Wiemer, Wolfgang Linz and
Bernward A. Schölkens

Aventis Pharma Deutschland GmbH, Disease Groups Research, Building H821, D-65926 Frankfurt/Main, Germany

Introduction

The endothelium is an important target organ of angiotensin converting enzyme (ACE) inhibitors. Within these monolayered cells establishing the interface between blood and vasculature, a complex signal transduction machinery is the basis for a major role of ACE inhibition in the regulation of vascular homoestasis. This chapter will focus on the endothelial aspects of ACE-inhibition, on its interaction with components of the kallikrein-kinin system.

ACE degrades bradykinin and kallidin, the N-terminal elongated form of bradykinin (BK). Inhibition of ACE leads to accumulation of both kinins with a subsequent stimulation of endothelial B_2 kinin receptors causing the synthesis and release of vasodilator substances such as endothelium-derived hyperpolarizing factor (EDHF) [1], prostacyclin and nitric oxide (NO) [2]. In addition to this basic mechanism, recent results indicate a direct interaction between ACE inhibitors and/or ACE and B_2 kinin receptors amplifying this signaling pathway. Furthermore, mutual feedback inhibition between ACE and NO by transcriptional and post-transcriptional mechanisms tightly control the whole cascade.

Effect of ACE inhibitors on endothelial B_2 kinin receptor activation and sequestration

The relative contribution of NO to the dilator response of BK and ACE inhibitors was shown in numerous investigations with isolated ischaemic rat hearts [3–5] and isolated intact blood vessels from different species including coronary microvessels and large arteries from the dog [6], and microvessels from failing human hearts [7]. The significance of the endothelium in the action of BK and ACE inhibitors could be demonstrated in experiments in cultured endothelial cells from different sized vessels and different species [2,

8–10]. In these studies ACE inhibition, like exogenously added BK, led to an enhanced accumulation of endothelial cyclic GMP, which can be considered as an index for NO synthesis and release [11].

Studies with isolated porcine [12], canine [13], bovine and human coronary arteries [14, 15] provide increasing experimental evidence that ACE inhibitors not only facilitate the accumulation of locally formed kinins but also directly affect endothelial B_2 kinin receptor signaling which results in an enhanced vascular response to BK. Two mechanisms are currently being discussed. First, ACE inhibitors might directly bind to, and modulate in an ACE-independent manner, B_2 kinin receptors. Indeed, ACE inhibitors were able to amplify the BK-induced contraction and to directly increase the tone in endothelium-denuded rabbit jugular veins, which lacked measurable ACE activity. Moreover, ramiprilat markedly enhanced the constrictor effect in the presence of an ACE-resistant B_2 kinin receptor agonist [16, 17]. These effects were blocked by the specific B_2 kinin receptor antagonist icatibant. Similarly, *ex vivo* data [18] showed that a 12 week long treatment with an ACE inhibitor potentiated and even unmasked the dilator actions of BK in mesenteric arterial rings of spontaneously hypertensive rats. Second, beyond this assumption of a direct interaction between ACE inhibitor and B_2 kinin receptor are data providing evidence for an ACE inhibitor-induced transmembrane interaction between ACE and and the B_2 kinin receptor. Only in chinese hamster ovary (CHO) cells co-transfected with both the human ACE and B_2 kinin receptor could it be demonstrated that ACE inhibitors augmented the release of signal transduction products by BK independent of inhibiting the degradation of BK [19]. In CHO cells transfected with the B_2 kinin receptor alone no effect of the ACE inhibitor was observed. Stimulation of native porcine endothelial cells with BK resulted in the time-dependent sequestration of the B_2 kinin receptors in caveolin-rich membranes, assessed by [^{3}H] bradykinin binding and immunoprecipation. In contrast, pre-treatment with the ACE inhibitor ramiprilat significantly attenuated this process increasing the amount of B_2 kinin receptors in membranes lacking the caveoleae marker protein [20]. This seemed to be distinct from BK degradation, since [^{3}H]-BK binding was not influenced in the presence of an inhibitory concentration of a synthetic ACE substrate, which blocked the kininase-II activity of ACE. Therefore, it was suggested that ACE inhibitors stabilize the B_2 kinin receptor in a G-protein coupled active form, thereby preventing and or reversing its BK-induced sesquestration to caveolae [21] prior to internalization. A recent report extended these oberservations by showing that the ACE inhibitor enalaprilat potentiated the effect of BK in cells expressing a mutant ACE with a single N-domain active site [22]. Thus by reacting with this site of ACE, enalaprilat induced a close interaction between ACE and the B_2 kinin receptor leading to a resensitization of BK receptors and potentiation of the BK effect, respectively.

Inverse relationship between ACE expression or activity and the endothelial NO pathway

The ACE-inhibitor-mediated endothelial NO release is under mutual feedback control. Regulation of ACE expression or activity by NO was examined by several investigators. Chronic inhibition of endothelial NO synthase (eNOS) led to an upregulation of cardiac and vascular ACE activity [23, 24]. In addition to this effect on ACE-expression, it was demonstrated that NO endogenously released or NO-donating compounds were capable of directly inhibiting the activity of purified ACE or the conversion of angiotensin-I to angiotensin-II (ANG-II) [25]. This inverse relationship between ACE inhibition and NO was also found in hypertensive rats; long-term ACE inhibition of vascular and cardiac ACE activity was associated with an upregulated eNOS expression and increased vascular NO release [26, 27]. This ACE inhibition-mediated modulation of eNOS expression could also be demonstrated in cultured endothelial cells indicating an autocrine effect. In primary cultured bovine aortic endothelial cells incubated for 36 h with the ACE inhibitor ramiprilat, an approximately 2-fold increase in eNOS expression could be observed, which was sustained for at least 72 h of incubation [28]. This increase in eNOS expression was accompanied by an enhanced production of cyclic GMP after maximal stimulation with the calcium ionophore A23187. In comparison, transforming growth factor-β1 (TGF-β1) which is known as a "standard" for induction of eNOS [31], led to a 2 to 4-fold increase of eNOS expression after 36 and 72 h of incubation, respectively, and in parallel to an increase in endothelial cyclic GMP production.

Taken together, these observations provided evidence for a close feedback regulation between eNOS expression and/or activity and tissue ACE expression and/or activity. Surprisingly, in cultured human endothelial cells, enhancement of cyclic GMP formation by atrial natriuretic factor, phosphodiesterase inhibition or addition of 8-bromo-cyclic GMP, was accompanied by an increased ACE activity [30]. These findings indicate that NO and cyclic GMP may modulate ACE expression and/or activity by different mechanisms.

Dissimilarities but also similarities in the endothelial mechanisms of ACE inhibitors and ANG-II-subtype AT$_1$-receptor antagonists

Both ACE inhibitors and ANG-II-subtype AT$_1$-receptor antagonists (AT$_1$ antagonists) interfere with the renin-angiotensin-system at different steps in the signaling cascade. AT$_1$ antagonists act by a specific blockade of the ANG-II–subtype AT$_1$-receptor whereas ACE inhibitors inhibit ANG-II formation but also degradation of kinins. Therefore, it was concluded that the cardioprotective effects of AT$_1$ antagonists might deliver a better, kinin-independent therapy with less potential kinin-mediated side effects. However, recent evidences question this initial view.

Blockade of AT_1 receptors increases plasma renin and ANG-II in rats [31] and in healthy volunteers [32]. Specific blockade of the ANG-II-subtype AT_1-receptor leaves the ANG-II-subtype AT_2-receptor unopposed to the increaesed levels of ANG-II. This receptor subtype could be demonstrated in fetus, brain, myometrium, kidney, lung and heart (for a review see [33]) and seems to deliver a counterregulation against the AT_1 receptor-mediated effects of ANG-II. Beside influences on behaviour, knockout-mice for this receptor subtype displayed also an elevated blood pressure and a hyperresponsiveness to ANG-II pressor action [34]. The signal transduction activated by the AT_2 receptor subtype include G_i-protein-mediated activation of tyrosine and serine/threonine phosphatase with a subsequent modulation of potassium and calcium channels. Additionally, via an unknown signal transduction pathway, this receptor subtype seems to be also coupled to endothelial kinin synthesis and subsequent increases in NO/cGMP explain best its vasodilatory effect. In cultivated bovine endothelial cells ANG-II concentration-dependently stimulated cyclic GMP production and enhanced the release of endogenous kinins [35]. These effect was blocked by icatibant as well as the NO synthase inhibitor L-N^G-nitroarginine (L-NNA) [36]. Icatibant and L-NNA also blocked the ANG-II-induced production of NO, assessed by nitrite release, in coronary microvessels and large coronary arteries of the dog [37]. The protection of isolated rat hearts against postischaemic reperfusion injuries in the presence of an AT_1 antagonist and a low (10^{-10} mol/l) concentration of ANG-II was abolished again by L-NNA and icatibant [38].

The hypothesis of subsequent activation of ANG-II-subtype AT_2 receptors and increased kinin synthesis as a consequence solely of AT_1 antagonism was recently prove in experimental models of heart failure and hypertension. When two months after myocardial infarction rats were treated for two months with an ACE inhibitor or AT_1 antagonist, the decrease in left ventricular end-diastolic and end-systolic volume observed under AT_1 antagonist could be blocked by an AT_2 receptor antagonist and attenuated by a specific B_2 kinin receptor antagonist [39]. In a pig model of acute myocardioal infarction, pre-treatment with an AT_2 receptor antagonist, a bradykinin receptor antagonist or the cyclooxygenase inhibitor *per se* did not affect infarct size but abolished the reduction achieved by a specific AT_1 antagonist [40]. Similarly, in isolated rat hearts, pre- and postischemic treatment with an AT_1 antagonist protected against acute ischemia and reperfusion injury by a bradykinin dependent mechanism [41]. In the stroke prone strain of spontaneously hypertensive rats, the effect of AT_1 antagonist on aortic cyclic GMP could be attenuated by B_2-receptor blockade as well as NO synthase inhibition [42]. Overall these recent findings indicate that AT_1 antagonism is not a completely kinin-independent therapeutic principle. In contrast to ACE inhibitors AT_1 antagonists increase kinin synthesis but do not decrease kinin degradation. The final outcome of increased amounts of kinins and subsequent activation of endothelium-derived NO synthesis seems to be similar. Additionally, it should be noted that AT_1 antagonists, in contrast to ACE inhibitors, do not induce a crosstalk between

ACE and the B$_2$ kinin receptor. Although levels of ANG-II are increased under AT$_1$ receptor blockade, ANG-II *per se* is neither a substrate nor an inhibitor of ACE [43].

Clinically, the involvement of kinins in the mode of action of AT$_1$ antagonists will be difficult to prove or disprove. Of particular interest are reports of cough and angioedema among the first reports of adverse drug reactions from treatment with AT$_1$ antagonists. The clinical characterisitics were remarkably similar to those seen with ACE inhibitors [44]. It was initially expected that these complications of ACE inhibitor therapy are due to inhibition of kinin degradation and would be avoided with AT$_1$ receptor antagonists.

Conclusion

Our knowledge on the mode of actions of ACE-inhibitors is still increasing. In contrast to a rather simplified view at the beginning of the development of ACE inhibitors, more complex mechanisms are currently being discovered and discussed (Fig. 1). In particular the endothelium, an important interface between blood and vasculature, seems to deliver a biological milieu for a crosstalk between ACE, kinins, B$_2$ kinin receptors and NO. Among the recently discovered mechanisms of ACE inhibitors, the modulation of the B$_2$ kinin receptor sequestration and eNOS expression amplify the ACE inhibitor-stimu-

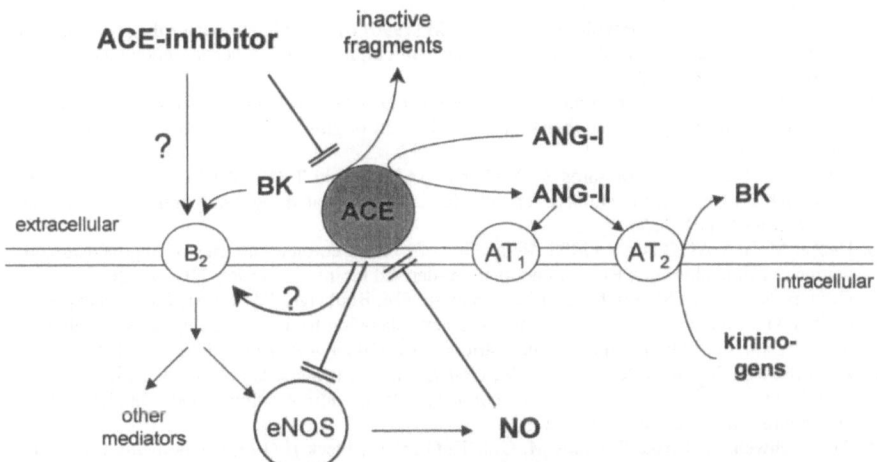

Figure 1. Crosstalk between ACE, kinins and NO in endothelial cells. Inhibition of angiotensin converting enzyme (ACE) leads to accumulation of kinins (BK), stimulation of the B$_2$ kinin receptor (B$_2$), activation of the endothelial constitutive nitric oxide synthase (eNOS) and a subsequent release of nitric oxide. The components of this system are connected in a complex network of mutual interactions, which are described in detail in the text. In contrast to ACE-inhibition, blockade of the ANG-II-subtype AT$_1$-receptor (AT$_1$) directs ANG-II to the ANG-II-subtype AT$_2$-receptor (AT$_2$), which is coupled with the formation of kinins.

lated synthesis and release of NO. In their endothelial mode of action, ACE inhibitors and AT_1 antagonists lead to increased amounts of endothelial kinin via different mechanisms. In contrast to AT_1 antagonists, ACE inhibitors offer the additional advantage of B_2 kinin receptor modulation.

References

1 Mombouli J-V, Vanhoutte PM (1996) Kinins and endothelial control of vascular smooth muscle. *Annu Rev Pharmacol Toxicol* 35: 679–705
2 Wiemer G, Schölkens BA, Becker RHA, Busse R (1991) Ramiprilat enhances endothelial autacoid formation by inhibiting breakdown of endothelium-derived bradykinin. *Hypertension* 18: 558–563
3 Linz W, Wiemer G, Schölkens BA (1992) ACE-inhibition induces NO-formation in cultured bovine aortic endothelial cells and protects isolated ischaemic rat hearts. *J Mol Cell Cardiol* 24: 909–919
4 Parratt JR (1994) Cardioprotection by angiotensin converting enzyme inhibitors-the experimental evidence. *Cardiovasc Res* 28: 183–189
5 Liu Y-H, Yang X-P, Sharov VG, Sigmon DH, Sabbah HN, Carretero OA (1996) Paracrine systems in the cardioprotective effect of angiotensin converting enzyme inhibitors on myocardial ischaemia/reperfusion injury in rats. *Hypertension* 27: 7–13
6 Busse R, Fleming I, Hecker M (1993) Endothelium-derived bradykinin: Implications for angiotensin-converting enzyme-inhibitor therapy. *J Cardiovasc Pharmcol* 22 (suppl 5): S31–S36
7 Kichuk MR, Seyedi N, Zhang X, Marboe CC, Michler RE, Addonizio LJ, Kaley G, Nasjletti A, Hintze TH (1996) Regulation of nitric oxide production in human coronary microvessels and the contribution of local kinin formation. *Circulation* 94: 44–51
8 Brotherton AFA (1986) Induction of prostacyclin biosynthesis is closely associated with guanosine 3',5'-cyclic monophosphate accumulation in cultured human endothelium. *J Clin Invest* 78: 1253–1260
9 Schini VB, Boulanger C, Regoli D, Vanhoutte PM (1990) Bradykinin stimulates the production of cyclic GMP via activation of B_2 kinin receptors in cultured porcine aortic endothelial cells. *J Pharmacol Exp Ther* 252: 581–585
10 Wohlfart P, Dedio J, Wirth K, Schölkens BA, Wiemer G (1997) Different B_1 kinin receptor expression and pharmacology in endothelial cells of different origins and species. *J Pharmacol Exper Ther* 280: 1109–1116
11 Wiemer G, Pierchala B, Mesaros S, Schölkens BA, Malinski T (1996) Direct measurement of nitric oxide release from cultured endothelial cells stimulated by bradykinin or ramiprilat. *Endothelium* 4: 119–125
12 Hecker M, Bara AT, Busse R (1993) Relaxation of isolated coronary arteries by angiotensin-converting enzyme inhibitors: Role of endothelium-derived kinins. *J Vasc Res* 30: 257–262
13 Desta B, Nakashima M, Kirchengast M, Vanhoutte PM, Boulanger CM (1994) Previous exposure to bradykinin unmasks an endothelium-dependent relaxation to the converting enzyme inhibitor trandolaprilat in isolated canine coronary arteries. *J Pharmacol Exp Ther* 272: 885–891
14 Auch-Schwelk W, Bossaller C, Claus M, Graf K, Gräfe M, Fleck E (1993) ACE inhibitors are endothelium dependent vasodilators of coronary arteries during submaximal stimulation with bradykinin. *Cardiovasc Res* 27: 312–317
15 Auch-Schwelk W, Duske E, Claus M, Graf K, Gräfe M, Fleck E (1995) Endothelium-mediated vasodilation during ACE inhibition. *Eur Heart J* 16 (suppl C): 59–65
16 Hecker M, Pörsti I, Bara AT, Busse R (1994) Potentiation by ACE inhibitors of the dilator response to bradykinin in the coronary microcirculation: interaction at the receptor level. *Brit J Pharmacol* 111: 238–244
17 Hecker M, Blaukat A, Bara AT, Müller-Esterl W, Busse R (1997) ACE inhibitor potentiation of bradykinin-induced venoconstriction. *Brit J Pharmacol* 121: 1475–1481
18 Hutri-Kähönen N, Pörsti I, Wu X, Tolvanen J-P, Sallinen K, Kähönen M (1997) Arterial responses to bradykinin after ramipril therapy in experimental hypertension. *Pharmacol Toxicol* 81: 190–196

19 Minshall RD, Tan F, Nakamura F, Rabito SF, Becker RP, Marcic B, Erdös EG (1997) Potentiation of the actions of bradykinin by angiotensin I-converting enzyme inhibitors. The role of expressed human bradykinin B_2 receptors and angiotensin I-converting enzyme in CHO cells. *Circ Res* 81: 848–856

20 Benzing T, Fleming I, Blaukat A, Müller-Esterl W, Busse R (1999) The ACE inhibitor ramiprilat interferes with the sequestration of the B_2 kinin receptor within the plasma membrane of native endothelial cells. *Circulation* 99: 2034–2040

21 Haasemann M, Cartaud J, Mueller-Esterl W, Dunia I (1998) Agonist-induced redistribution of bradykinin B_2 receptor in caveolae. *J Cell Sci* 111: 917–928

22 Marcic B, Deddish PA, Jackman HL, Erdös EG (1999) Enhancement of bradykinin and resensitization of its B_2 receptor. *Hypertension* 33: 835–843

23 Michel J-B, Xu Y, Blot S, Philippe M, Chatellier G (1996) Improved survival in rats administered N^G-nitro-L-arginine methyl ester due to converting enzyme inhibition. *J Cardiovasc Pharmacol* 28: 142–148

24 Takemoto M, Egashira K, Usui M, Numaguchi K, Tomita H, Tsutsui H, Shimokawa H, Sueshi K, Takeshita A (1997) Important role of tissue angiotensin-converting enzyme activity in the pathogenesis of coronary vascular and myocardial structural changes induced by long-term blockade of nitric oxide synthesis in rats. *J Clin Invest* 99: 278–287

25 Ackermann A, Fernandez-Alfonso MS, Sanchez de Rojas R, Ortega T, Paul M, Gonzalez C (1998) Modulation of angiotensin-converting enzyme by nitric oxide. *Brit J Pharmacol* 124: 291–298

26 Linz W, Jessen T, Becker RHA, Schölkens BA, Wiemer G (1997) Long-term ACE inhibition doubles lifespan of hypertensive rats. *Circulation* 96: 3164–3172

27 Wiemer G, Linz W, Hatrik S, Schölkens BA, Malinski T (1997) Angiotensin-converting enzyme inhibition alters nitric oxide and superoxide release in normotensive and hypertensive rats. *Hypertension* 30: 1183–1190

28 Linz W, Wohlfart P, Schölkens BA, Malinski T, Wiemer G (1999) Interactions among ACE, kinins and NO. *Cardiovasc Res* 43: 549–561

29 Inoue N, Venema RC, Sayegh HS, Ohara Y, Murphy TJ, Harrisson DG (1995) Molecular regulation of the bovine endothelial cell nitric oxide synthase by transforming growth factor-$\beta 1$. *Arterioscler Thromb Vasc Biol* 15: 1255–1261

30 Saijonmaa O, Fyrquist F (1998) Upregulation of angiotensin converting enzyme by atrial natriuretic peptide and cyclic GMP in human endothelial cells. *Cardiovasc Res* 40: 206–210

31 Campbell DJ, Kladis A, Valentjin AJ (1995) Effects of losartan on angiotensin and bradykinin peptides and angiotensin-converting enzyme. *J Cardiovasc Pharmacol* 6: 1043–1047

32 Hubner R, Hogemann AM, Sunzel M, Riddell JG (1997) Pharmacokinetics of candesartan after single and repeated doses of candesartan cilexetil in young and elderly healthy volunteers. *J Hum Hypertens* 11 (suppl 2): S19–25

33 Matsubara H (1998) Pathophysiological role of angiotensin II type 2 receptor in cardiovascular and renal diseases. *Circ Res* 83: 1182–1191

34 Hein L, Barsh GS, Pratt RE, Dzau VJ, Koblik BK (1995) Behavioral and cardiovascular effects of disrupting the angiotensin II type-2 receptor gene in mice. *Nature* 377: 744–747

35 Korth P, Fink E, Linz W, Schölkens BA, Wohlfart P, Wiemer G (1995) Angiotensin II receptor subtype-stimulated formation of endothelial cyclic GMP and prostacyclin is accompanied by an enhanced release of endogenous kinins. *Pharm Pharmacol Lett* 5: 124–127

36 Wiemer G, Schölkens BA, Busse R, Wagner A, Heitsch H, Linz W (1993) The functional role of angiotensin II-subtype AT_2-receptors in endothelial cells and isolated ischaemic rat hearts. *Pharm Pharmacol Lett* 3: 24–27

37 Seyedi N, Xu X, Nasjletti A, Hintze TH (1995) Coronary kinin generation mediates nitric oxide release after angiotensin receptor stimulation. *Hypertension* 26: 164–170

38 Wiemer G, Schölkens BA, Wagner A, Heitsch H, Linz W (1993) The possible role of angiotensin II subtype AT_2 receptors in endothelial cells and isolated ischaemic rat hearts. *J Hypertension* 11 (suppl 5):S234–S235

39 Liu YH, Yang XP, Sharov VG, Nass O, Sabbah HN, Peterson E, Carretero OA (1997) Effects of angiotensin-converting enzyme inhibitors and agniotensin II type 1 receptor antagonists in rats with heart failure. *J Clin Invest* 99: 1926–1935

40 Jalowy A, Schulz R, Dörge H, Behrends M, Heusch G (1998) Infarct size reduction by AT_1-receptor blockade through a signal cascade of AT_2-receptor activation, bradykinin and prostaglandins in pigs. *J Amer Coll Cardiol* 32: 1787–1796

41 Zhu P, Zaugg CE, Hornstein PS, Allegrini PR, Buser PT (1999) Bradykinin dependent cardioprotective effects of losartan against ischemia and reperfusion in rat hearts. *J Cardiovasc Pharmacol*
   33: 785–790
42 Gohlke P, Pees C, Unger T (1998) AT_2 receptor stimulation increases aortic cyclic GMP in SHRSP
   by a kinin-dependent mechanism. *Hypertension* 31 (part 2): 349–355
43 Deddish PA, Marcic B, Jackman HL, Wang H-Z, Skidgel RA, Erdös EG (1998) N-domain-spe-
   cific substrate and C-domain inhibitors of angiotensin-converting enzyme. Angiotensin-(1-7) and
   keto-ACE. *Hypertension* 31: 912–917
44 Mathew T, Desmond P, Isaacs D, Lander C, Shenfield G, Wainwright D, Wing L (1999)
   Angiotensin II receptor antagonists – new drugs with some old problems and some new problems.
   Aust Adverse Drug React Bull 18 (1): 1–3

ACE Inhibitors
ed. by P. D'Orléans-Juste and G.E. Plante
© 2001 Birkhäuser Verlag/Switzerland

Interactions between the ACE and the endothelin pathway

Rob L. Hopfner, J. Robert McNeill and Venkat Gopalakrishnan

Department of Pharmacology and the Cardiovascular Risk Factor Reduction Unit (CRFRU), College of Medicine, University of Saskatchewan, Saskatoon, SK, Canada

Angiotensin-endothelin interactions: an emerging paradigm

Endothelin-1 (ET-1) is released from endothelial cells (EC) following gene activation of preproET mRNA and the subsequent proteolytic processing into biologically active peptide [1]. ET-1 activates ET_B receptors on EC, promoting the release of endothelium-derived relaxing factor (EDRF), and ET_A and ET_B receptors on vascular smooth muscle cells (VSMC), promoting events coupled to both vasoconstriction and growth [2]. Activation of ET_A/ET_B receptors by ET-1 results in activation of the effector enzyme, phospholipase C (PLC) through a G_q-coupled receptor with the subsequent production of the hydrolytic products 1,4,5 inositol-trisphosphate (IP_3) and diacylglycerol (DAG) [2]. These mediators subsequently promote $[Ca^{2+}]_i$ release from sarcoplasmic reticulum (SR) stores and activate protein kinase C (PKC) respectively.

In 1989, Emori et al. first demonstrated the ability of thrombin, arginine vasopressin (AVP) and angiotensin II (Ang II) to enhance ET-1 release from cultured bovine EC [3]. Subsequent studies demonstrated that PKC activation, $[Ca^{2+}]_i$ mobilization and ET-1 gene expression are required to evoke this effect [4, 5]. Similar effects of Ang II were also demonstrated in cultured VSMC [6], mesangial cells [7], cardiac myocytes [8], endocardial [9], and retinal EC [10]. Several *in vitro* studies have also shown that Ang II modulates ET receptors [11–13] and activation of ET converting enzyme (ECE) [14]. Conversely, there is also evidence that ET-1 might regulate the renin-angiotensin system (RAS)-indicating potential Ang II-dependent actions of ET-1 [15–18].

In rabbit aortic rings, inclusion of the ET_A selective antagonist, BQ123, in the incubation medium, shifted the concentration–vasoconstriction response curves to Ang II to the right, without binding to Ang II receptors or affecting Ang II-evoked IP_3 production [19]. This provided the first evidence that ET-1 may be involved in a functional response to Ang II. Our laboratory later confirmed an ET-1 component to Ang II evoked vasoconstriction *in vitro*, and demonstrated regional, vascular bed differences in the dependence of ET-1 on the Ang II response [20, 21]. Vasoconstriction to Ang II in aorta was least dependent, mesenteric artery partially dependent, and tail artery was entirely dependent on ET-1 release from the vascular endothelium. Such *in vitro* functional studies were the impetus for further *in vivo* and other targeted studies investigating the physiological and pathophysiological relevance of this interaction.

Functional relevance and physiological significance

Blood pressure regulation

An interaction between Ang II and ET-1 in blood pressure regulation was first noted in a report by Yoshida et al. (1992) who demonstrated that sub-pressor doses of ET-1 and Ang II, but not ET-1 and norepinephrine, work synergistically to raise blood pressure in rats [22]. Our laboratory was the first to demonstrate that the hemodynamic response to acute infusions of low dose, but not high dose, Ang II in spontaneously hypertensive rats (SHR) and normotensive Wistar–Kyoto (WKY) rats could be blunted by co-infusion with the non-selective ET_A/ET_B antagonist, bosentan [23]. Interestingly, the ET dependence of the response to low dose Ang II was much more pronounced in the SHR group. Subsequent reports demonstrated that increases in blood pressure resulting from long-term Ang II infusion in rats could be blunted by an ET_A selective antagonist, (i) in conjunction with improvement in endothelial function [24]; (ii) with a reduction in tissue ET-1 content [25]; and (iii) with correction of vasoconstrictor responsiveness to a variety of vasoactive agents [26]. Herizi et al. (1998) recently demonstrated that mixed ET_A/ET_B blockade prevented increases in blood pressure to ten days of Ang II infusion in conjunction with prevention of changes in renal blood flow, albuminuria, heart weight index, and carotid media thickness [27]. Thus, several lines of evidence indicate ET-1 dependence in both the acute and chronic hemodynamic actions of Ang II, as well as in the sequelae resulting from the deleterious hemodynamic actions of Ang II.

While the pharmacological actions of ACE inhibitors have been extensively characterized, there is a paucity of information on the role of ET-1 in hemodynamic responses to ACE inhibitors. One study demonstrated the ability of captopril to reduce plasma ET-1 levels in essential hypertensives [28]. It has been hypothesized that hyperinsulinemia might promote increases in blood pressure through increased ET-1 production [29]. Type II diabetic men treated for one week with captopril were shown to exhibit reduced insulin-induced increments in plasma ET-1 levels, along with enhanced glucose uptake [30]. Moreover, both spontaneous and insulin-stimulated ET-1 production were later shown to be inhibited by captopril in both cultured human EC and after a one week treatment period in normal and hypertensive humans [31]. These studies demonstrate an important interaction between ACE and the ET system in hyperinsulinemic states of potential relevance to the regulation of blood pressure. Conversely, ACE inhibition was also shown to prevent hypertension caused by long-term administration of ET-1 in rats [32]. These results indicate that Ang II might also contribute to the hemodynamic actions of ET-1.

Cardiac function

ET-1 has well-established actions on cardiac function. Ito et al. (1993) first demonstrated that Ang II-evoked cardiomyocyte hypertrophy could be blocked by ET receptor antagonists and antisense oligonucleotides to preproET mRNA [8]. Subsequent studies indicated that the cardiac trophic actions of Ang II *in vitro* involves synthesis of ET-1 in fibroblasts, and the subsequent paracrine activation of protein synthesis in cardiac myocytes [33, 34].

It is uncertain whether ACE inhibitors modulate ET-1 in cardiac physiology. A single oral dose of captopril given to patients with congestive heart failure (CHF) reduced RAS overactivation, but did not affect plasma concentrations of ET-1 [35]. Another study demonstrated that administration of captopril failed to affect plasma ET-1 levels during thrombolysis and reperfusion post-myocardial infarction (MI) [36]. However, the same group in a later study has demonstrated that treatment with captopril *actually* decreased plasma ET-1 levels in post-MI patients recovering from acute and sub-acute stages of MI [37]. Moreover, 12 weeks of ACE inhibitor treatment overcame elevated ET-1 levels in patients with congestive heart failure (CHF) [38] and seven days of treatment with an ACE inhibitor attenuated elevated ET-1 levels in plasma and tissues in a dog model of CHF [39]. Thus, the available data appears to indicate that modulation of the ET system by ACE inhibitors in cardiac disease is a process that is slow to develop.

Renal function

Using a monoclonal antibody to ET-1, Bakris et al. (1993) first demonstrated that the mitogenic effect of Ang II in human mesangial cells is partially mediated by ET-1 [40]. Matrix protein synthesis and mesangial cell growth induced by Ang II and ET-1 were later shown to involve PKC, TGF-β expression, and the release of one peptide by the other [41]. It was later shown that two weeks of Ang II infusion in rats promoted a three-fold increase in renal ET-1 content [14].

In conjunction with other beneficial renal actions, ACE inhibitors have been shown to: i) reduce ET-1 content in mesangial cells [42]; ii) selectively decrease ET-1 mRNA levels in glomeruli of diabetic rats [43]; iii) decrease renal preproET-1 gene transcription, ET_A receptor expression, and ET-1 protein levels in a normotensive model of immune-complex nephritis [44]; iv) diminish elevated renal ET-1 expression and synthesis in uninephrectomized SHR [45]; and v) reduce tissue ET-1 content in various blood vessels of a rat remnant kidney model [46]. Thus, considerable evidence indicates that ACE inhibitors modulate ET-1 production in renal tissue across a wide range of experimental animal models of renal disease.

ACE inhibitors and ET-1: mechanistic considerations

As can be seen from the results presented above, ACE inhibitors are used widely as a means of modulating the RAS in studying the role of Ang II-evoked modulation of ET-1. However, the mechanism behind such actions of ACE inhibitors is subject to debate. Observations that ACE not only catalyzes formation of Ang II, but also degrades bradykinin [47], a potent, anti-mitogenic and vasodilatory mediator, provided the first evidence that ACE inhibitors may be acting through a pathway independent of blockade of Ang II production. The observation that enzymes other than ACE are also capable of catalyzing conversion of Ang I to Ang II [48] and that Ang II plasma [49] and tissue [50, 51] levels are restored after long-term ACE inhibitor therapy provide further evidence in support of this hypothesis. This conviction, interestingly, may also apply to the role of ACE inhibitors in modulating ET-1 production (Fig. 1). *Firstly*, a decrease in hemodynamic shear stress secondary to blood pressure reductions during ACE inhibitor therapy would be expected to attenuate ET-1 production in the vascular endothelium [52]. *Secondly*, and perhaps more importantly, potentiation of bradykinin may regulate ET-1 production and action. Both bradykinin and EDRF (whose release is stimulated by bradykinin) are known to potently inhibit ET-1 release [53, 54]. A well-designed study by Momose et al. (1993) using bradykinin antagonists and inhibitors of nitric oxide synthase (NOS) clearly indicated that ACE inhibitors potentiate bradykinin in EC, consequently stimulating EDRF production, subsequently inhibiting ET-1 release [55]. Another recent study demonstrated that ACE inhibitors suppress endogenous ET-1 secretion, through both Ang II inhibition and bradykinin potentiation, resulting in improved coronary function and stabilization of cardiac rhythm after ischemia in a rat model of reperfusion arrythmia [56]. In the final analysis, it appears that ACE inhibitors likely affect ET-1 release and action through multiple, independent mechanisms.

It should be noted that some studies fail to demonstrate an effect of ACE inhibition on ET-1 release and action. The observation that the hypotensive effect of a 30 min ACE inhibitor infusion were additive with those of an ET_A/ET_B antagonist in hypertensive dogs [57] suggested that the effects of ACE inhibitors are in fact independent of ET-1. Moreover, single dose captopril administration failed to affect plasma ET levels in patients with CHF [35] and patients undergoing thrombolysis and reperfusion post-MI [36]. However, it was later demonstrated that captopril decreased plasma ET-1 levels in the acute and sub-acute stages *after* MI [37] as well as after 12 weeks of treatment in CHF patients [38]. Thus, ACE inhibitors might modulate ET-1 production only after long-term treatment.

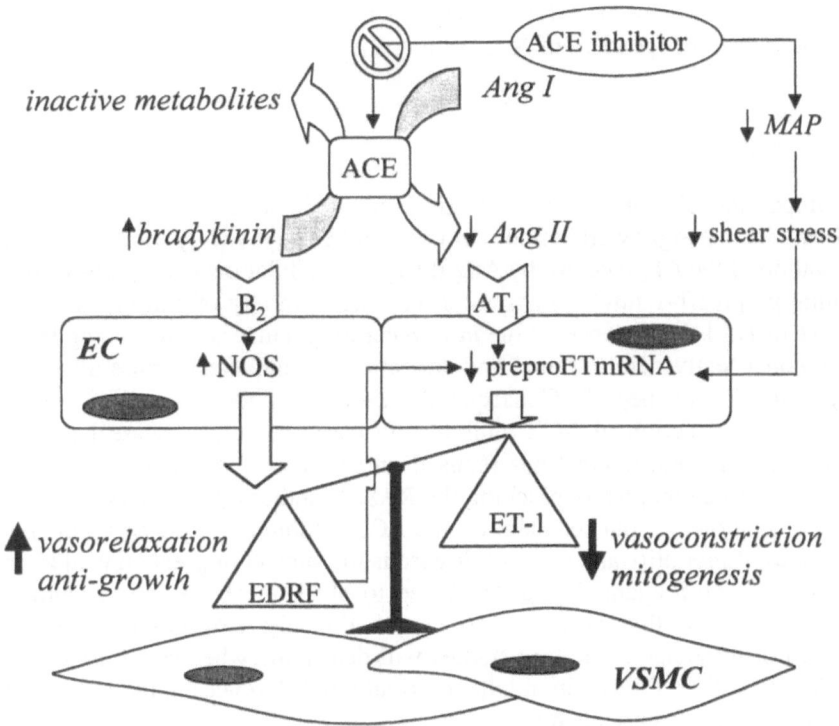

Figure 1. Effect of ACE inhibition on endothelial production and release of ET-1 and EDRF. ACE inhibition decreases processing of Ang I to Ang II, and inhibits the degradation of bradykinin, a potent vasodilatory and anti-growth promoting peptide. The former mechanism decreases Ang II production, attenuating AT₁ receptor-stimulated preproET mRNA induction and the latter would potentiate bradykinin, leading to increased nitric oxide synthase (NOS) activity and EDRF generation. Both mechanisms would consequently lead to reduced preproET mRNA induction. In addition, the hemo-dynamic actions of ACE inhibitors in lowering mean arterial pressure (MAP) might attenuate shear stress-induced ET-1 release. Thus, in the presence of ACE inhibition, the balance of endothelial mod-ulation of vascular smooth muscle tone would be tipped to favor vasodilatation and anti-growth effects. EC – endothelial cell; VSMC – vascular smooth muscle cell.

There is also some evidence that ACE inhibitors are capable of modulating responses to ET-1. Enalapril was shown to prevent both the hypertensive and renal vasoconstrictor response to ET-1 in humans [58]. In line with this, low dose enalaprilat infusion was shown to inhibit ET-1-evoked increases in fore-arm vascular resistance in humans [59]. Thus, not only do ACE inhibitors inhibit ET-1 release, but they also may be capable of inhibiting responses to exogenous ET-1 *in vivo*. It is likely that these actions are mediated through potentiation of bradykinin, since EDRF generated by bradykinin is capable of countering the physiological actions of ET-1 [53]. In support of this, ACE inhibition, but not AT₁ antagonism, was shown to prevent renal vasoconstric-tion evoked by short-term ET-1 infusion in rats [60], demonstrating that antagonism of the actions of ET-1 are caused by a mechanism unique to ACE inhibitors and independent of Ang II blockade.

Conclusions

An important role for ET-1 in mediating the cardiovascular actions of Ang II is being increasingly well defined. *In vitro* studies have firmly established that activation of the AT_1 receptor by Ang II triggers cellular events capable of regulating preproET-1 mRNA expression in a wide variety of cell types. Some degree of ET-1 dependence on the *in vivo* cardiovascular actions of Ang II has been consistently demonstrated and appears to be universal across all of the target sites for this peptide. Consequently, a role for modulation of ET-1 in the mechanism of action of ACE inhibitors in cardiovascular disease has been established. Recent interest has focused on the role of AT_1 antagonists as a means of more completely blocking the RAS. Whether these agents will meet the expectations set out for them by the ACE inhibitors on primary outcome measures of mortality and onset of disease is the subject of great clinical interest. Despite both agents being developed to block the RAS, it is becoming increasingly clear that there are distinct and clinically relevant unique actions of each of these agents. Future studies will determine whether differences in modulation of the ET system might contribute to differences in the pharmacological actions of these agents.

Acknowledgements
Referenced original work completed in the authors' (VG, JRMc) laboratories were supported by the Medical Research Council of Canada and the Heart and Stroke Foundation of Saskatchewan. Mr. Rob L. Hopfner is thankful to the Medical Research Council of Canada for the award of a Doctoral Research Scholarship.

References

1 Yanagisawa M, Kurihara H, Kimura S, Tomobe Y, Kobayashi M, Mitsui Y, Yazaki Y, Goto K, Masaki T (1988) A novel potent vasoconstrictor peptide produced by vascular endothelial cells. *Nature* 332: 411–415
2 Masaki T, Vane JR, Vanhoutte PM (1994) International Union of Pharmacology nomenclature of endothelin receptors. *Pharmacol Rev* 46: 137–142
3 Emori T, Hirata Y, Ohta K, Shichiri M, Marumo F (1989) Secretory mechanism of immunoreactive endothelin in cultured bovine endothelial cells. *Biochem Biophys Res Commun* 160: 93–100
4 Emori T, Hirata Y, Ohta K, Kanno K, Eguchi S, Imai T, Shichiri M, Marumo F (1991) Cellular mechanism of endothelin-1 release by angiotensin and vasopressin. *Hypertension* 18: 165–170
5 Imai T, Hirata Y, Emori T, Yanagisawa M, Masaki T, Marumo F (1992) Induction of endothelin-1 gene by angiotensin and vasopressin in endothelial cells. *Hypertension* 19: 753–757
6 Resink TJ, Hahn AW, Scott-Burden T, Powell J, Weber E, Buhler FR (1990) Inducible endothelin mRNA expression and peptide secretion in cultured human vascular smooth muscle cells. *Biochem Biophys Res Commun* 168: 1303–1310
7 Kohno M, Horio T, Ikeda M, Yokokawa K, Fukui T, Yasunari K, Kurihara N, Takeda T (1992) Angiotensin II stimulates endothelin-1 secretion in cultured rat mesangial cells. *Kidney Int* 42: 860–866

8 Ito H, Hirata Y, Tanaka M, Tsujino M, Koike A, Nogami A, Murumo F, Hiroe M (1993) Endothelin-1 is an autocrine/paracrine factor in the mechanism of angiotensin II induced hypertrophy in cultured rat cardiomyocytes. *J Clin Invest* 92: 398–403

9 Chua BH, Chua CC, Diglio CA, Siu BB (1993) Regulation of endothelin-1 mRNA by angiotensin II in rat heart endothelial cells. *Biochim Biophys Acta* 1178: 201–206

10 Higgins RD, Hendricks-Munoz KD, Caines VV, Gerrets RP, Rifkin DB (1998) Hyperoxia stimulates endothelin-1 secretion from endothelial cells; modulation by captopril and nifedipine. *Curr Eye Res* 17: 487–493

11 Roubert P, Gillard V, Plas P, Guillon JM, Chabrier PE, Braquet P (1989) Angiotensin II and phorbol esters potently down-regulate endothelin binding sites in vascular smooth muscle cells. *Biochem Biophys Res Commun* 164: 809–815

12 Kanno K, Hirata Y, Tsujino M, Imai T, Shichiri M, Ito H, Marumo F (1993) Up-regulation of ET_B receptor subtype mRNA by angiotensin II in rat cardiomyocytes. *Biochem Biophys Res Commun* 194: 1282–1287

13 Hatakeyama H, Miyamori I, Tamagishi S, Takeda Y, Takeda R, Yamamoto H (1994) Angiotensin II up-regulates the expression of type A endothelin receptor in human vascular smooth muscle cells. *Biochem Mol Biol Int* 34: 127–134

14 Barton M, Shaw S, d'Uscio LV, Moreau P, Luscher TF (1997) Angiotensin II increases vascular and renal endothelin-1 and functional endothelin converting enzyme activity *in vivo*: Role of ET_A receptors for endothelin regulation. *Biochem Biophys Res Commun* 238: 861–865

15 Goetz KL, Wang BC, Madwed JB, Zhu JL, Leadley RJ (1988) Cardiovsacular, renal, and endocrine responses to intravenous endothelin in conscious dogs. *Amer J Physiol* 255: R1064–R1068

16 Kawaguchi H, Sawa H, Yasuda H (1990) Endothelin stimulates angiotensin I to angiotensin II conversion in cultured pulmonary artery endothelial cells. *J Mol Cell Cardiol* 22: 839–842

17 Rakugi H, Tabuchi Y, Nakamura M, Nagano M, Higashimori K, Mikami H, Ogihara T (1990) Endothelin activates the vascular renin-angiotensin system in rat mesenteric arteries. *Biochem Int* 21: 867–872

18 Moroi M, Fukazawa M, Ishikawa M, Aikawa J, Namiki A, Yamaguchi T (1996) Effect of endothelin on angiotensin converting enzyme activity in cultured vascular smooth muscle cells. *Gen Pharmacol* 27: 463–465

19 Webb ML, Dickinson KE, Delaney CL, Liu EC, Serafino R, Cohen RB, Monshizadegan H, Moreland S (1992) The endothelin receptor antagonist, BQ123, inhibits angiotensin II induced contractions in rabbit aorta. *Biochem Biophys Res Commun* 185: 887–892

20 Chen L, McNeill JR, Wilson TW, Gopalakrishnan V (1995) Heterogeneity in vascular smooth muscle responsiveness to angiotensin II. Role of endothelin. *Hypertension* 26: 83–88

21 Chen L, McNeill JR, Wilson TW, Gopalakrishnan V (1995) Differential effects of phosphoramidon on contractile responses to angiotensin II in rat blood vessels. *Brit J Pharmacol* 114: 1599–1604

22 Yoshida K, Yasujima M, Kohzuki M, Kanazawa M, Yoshinaga K, Abe K (1992) Endothelin-1 augments pressor responses to angiotensin II infusion in rats. *Hypertension* 20: 292–297

23 Balakrishnan SM, Wang HD, Gopalakrishnan V, Wilson TW, McNeill JR (1996) Effect of an endothelin antagonist on hemodynamic responses to angiotensin II. *Hypertension* 28: 806–809

24 d'Uscio LV, Moreau P, Shaw S, Takase H, Barton M, Luscher TF (1997) Effects of chronic ETA receptor blockade in angiotensin II induced hypertension. *Hypertension* 29: 435–441

25 d'Uscio LV, Shaw S, Barton M, Luscher TF (1998) Losartan but not verapamil inhibits angiotensin II induced tissue endothelin-1 increase: role of blood pressure and endothelial function. *Hypertension* 31: 1305–1310

26 Rajagopalan S, Laursen JB, Borthayre A, Kurz S, Keiser J, Haleen S, Giaid A, Harrison DG (1997) Role for endothelin-1 in angiotensin II mediated hypertension. *Hypertension* 30: 29–34

27 Herizi A, Jover B, Bouriquet N, Mimran A (1998) Prevention of the cardiovascular and renal effects of angiotensin II by endothelin blockade. *Hypertension* 31: 10–14

28 Uemasa J, Munemura C, Fujihara M, Kawasaki H (1994) Inhibition of plasma endothelin-1 concentration by captopril in patients with essential hypertension. *Clin Nephrol* 41: 150–152

29 Oliver FJ, de la Rubia G, Feener EP, Lee M-E, Loeken MR, Shiba T, Quetermous T, King GL (1991) Stimulation of endothelin-1 gene expression by insulin in endothelial cells. *J Biol Chem* 266: 23,251–23,256

30 Ferri C, Laurenti O, Bellini C, Faldetta MR, Properzi G, Santucci A, de Mattia G (1995)

Circulating endothelin-1 levels in lean non-insulin dependent diabetic patients. Influence of ACE inhibition. *Amer J Hypertens* 8: 40–47

31 Desideri G, Ferri C, Bellini C, De Mattia G, Santucci A (1997) Effects of ACE inhibition on spontaneous and insulin stimulated endothelin-1 secretion: *in vitro* and *in vivo* studies. *Diabetes* 46: 81–86

32 Mortensen LH, Fink GD (1992) Captopril prevents chronic hypertension produced by infusion of endothelin-1 in rats. *Hypertension* 19: 676–680

33 Ponicke K, Heinroth-Hoffman I, Becker K, Brodde OE (1997) Trophic effect of angiotensin II in neonatal rat cardiomyocytes: role of endothelin-1 and non-myocyte cells. *Brit J Pharmacol* 121: 118–124

34 Gray MO, Long CS, Kalinyak JE, Li HT, Karliner JS (1998) Angiotensin II stimulates cardiac myocyte hypertrophy via paracrine release of TGF-beta 1 and endothelin-1 from fibroblasts. *Cardiovasc Res* 40: 352–363

35 Grenier O, Pousset F, Isnard R, Kalotka H, Carayon A, Maistre G, Lechat P, Guerot C, Thomas D, Komajda M (1996) Captopril does not acutely modulate plasma endothelin-1 concentration in human congestive heart failure. *Cardiovasc Drug Therapy* 10: 561–565

36 DiPasquale P, Paterna S, Parrinello G, Bucca V, Cannizzaro S, Pipitone F, Maringhini G, Scalzo S, Licata G (1995) Captopril does not affect plasma endothelin-1 during thrombolysis and reperfusion. *Int J Cardiol* 51: 131–135

37 Di Pasquale P, Valdes L, Albano V, Bucca V, Scalzo S, Pieri D, Maringhini G, Paterna S (1997) Early captopril treatment reduces plasma endothelin concentrations in the acute and subacute phases of myocardial infarction: a pilot study. *J Cardiovasc Pharmacol* 29: 202–208

38 Gelatius-Jensen S, Wroblewski H, Emmeluth C, Bie P, Haunso S, Kastrup J (1996) Plasma endothelin in congestive heart failure: effect of the ACE inhibitor, fosinopril. *Cardiovasc Res* 32: 1148–1154

39 Clavell AL, Mattingly MT, Stevens TL, Nir A, Wright S, Aarhus LL, Heublein DM, Burnett JCJr, (1996) Angiotensin converting enzyme inhibition modulates endogenous endothelin in chronic canine thoracic inferior vena caval constriction. *J Clin Invest* 97: 1286–1292

40 Bakris GL, Re RN (1993) Endothelin modulates angiotensin II induced mitogenesis of human mesangial cells. *Amer J Physiol* 264: F937–F942

41 Gomez-Garre D, Ruiz-Ortega M, Ortego M, Largo R, Lopez-Armada MJ, Plaza JJ, Gonzalez E, Egido J (1996) Effects and interactions of endothelin-1 and angiotensin II on matrix protein expression and synthesis and mesangial cell growth. *Hypertension* 27: 885–892

42 Bakris GL, Bhandaru S, Akerstrom V, Re RN (1994) ACE inhibitor mediated attenuation of mesangial cell growth. A role for endothelin. *Amer J Hypertens* 7: 583–590

43 Fukui M, Nakamura T, Ebihara I, Makita Y, Osada S, Tomino Y, Koide H (1994) Effects of enalapril on endothelin-1 and growth factor gene expression in diabetic rat glomeruli. *J Lab Clin Med* 123: 763–768

44 Ruiz-Ortega M, Gomez-Garre D, Liu XH, Blanco J, Largo R, Egido J (1997) Quinapril decreses renal endothelin-1 expression and synthesis in a normotensive model of immune-complex nephritis. *J Amer Soc Nephrol* 8: 756–768

45 Largo R, Gomez-Garre D, Liu XH, Alonso J, Blanco J, Plaza JJ, Egido J (1997) Endothelin-1 upregulation in the kidney of uninephrectomized spontaneously hypertensive rats and its modification by the angiotensin converting enzyme inhibitor quinapril. *Hypertension* 29: 1178–1185

46 Lariviere R, Lebel M, Kingma I, Grose JH, Boucher D (1998) Effects of losartan and captopril on endothelin-1 production in blood vessels and glomeruli of rats with reduced renal mass. *Amer J Hypertens* 11: 989–997

47 Erdos EG (1990) Angiotensin I converting enzyme and the changes in our concepts through the years. Lewis K. Dahl memorial lecture. *Review Hypertension* 16: 363–370

48 Dzau VJ, Sasamura H, Hein L (1993) Heterogeneity of angiotensin synthetic pathways and receptor subtypes: physiological and pharmacological implications. *J Hypertension* 11: S13–S18

49 Timmermans PB, Wong PC, Chiu AT, Herblin WF, Benfield P, Carini DJ, Lee RJ, Wexler RR, Saye JA, Smith RD (1993) Angiotensin II receptors and angiotensin II receptor antagonists. *Pharmacol Rev* 45: 205–251

50 Urata H, Healy B, Stewart RW, Bumpus FM, Husain A (1990) Angiotensin II-forming pathways in normal and failing human hearts. *Circ Res* 66: 883–890

51 Wolny A, Clozel JP, Rein J, Mory P, Vogt P, Turino M, Kiowski W, Fischli W (1997) Functional and biochemical analysis of angiotensin II-forming pathways in the human heart. *Circ Res* 80:

219–227

52 Yoshizumi M, Kurihara H, Sugiyama T, Takaku F, Yanagisawa M, Masaki T, Yazaki Y (1989) Hemodynamic sheer stress stimulates endothelin production by cultured endothelial cells. *Biochem Biophys Res Commun* 161: 859–864

53 Boulanger C, Luscher TF (1990) Release of endothelin from the porcine aorta. *J Clin Invest* 85: 587–590

54 Yoshida H, Nakamura M (1992) Inhibition by angiotensin converting enzyme inhibitors of endothelin secretion from cultured human endothelial cells. *Life Sci* 50: PL195–PL200

55 Momose N, Fukuo K, Morimoto S, Ogihara T (1993) Captopril inhibits endothelin-1 secretion from endothelial cells through bradykinin. *Hypertension* 21: 921–924

56 Brunner F, Kukovetz WR (1996) Postischemic antiarrythmic effects of angiotensin converting enzyme inhibitors. Role of suppression of endogenous endothelin secretion. *Circulation* 94: 1752–1761

57 Donckier JE, Massart PE, Hodeige D, Van Mechelen H, Clozel JP, Laloux O, Ketelslegers JM, Charlier AA, Heyndickx GR (1997) Additional hypotensive effect of endothelin-1 receptor antagonism in hypertensive dogs under angiotensin converting enzyme inhibition. *Circulation* 96: 1250–1256

58 Kaasjager KA, Koomans HA, Rabelink TJ (1995) Effectiveness of enalapril *versus* nifedipine to antagonize blood pressure and the renal response to endothelin in humans. *Hypertension* 25: 620–625

59 Abernethy DR, Laurie N, Andrawis NS (1995) Local angiotensin-converting enzyme inhibition blunts endothelin-1-induced increase in forearm vascular resistance. *Clin Pharmacol* 58: 328–334

60 Banks RO (1990) Effects of endothelin on renal function in dogs and rats. *Amer J Physiol* 27: F775–F780

ACE Inhibitors
ed. by P. D'Orléans-Juste and G.E. Plante
© 2001 Birkhäuser Verlag/Switzerland

Evaluative and epidemiological approaches of ACE therapy

Maxime Lamarre-Cliche and Pierre Larochelle

Department of Medicine, Internal Medicine Service, Centre Hospitalier de l'Université de Montréal, Hôtel-Dieu, 3840 St.Urbain Street, Montreal, Quebec H2W 1T8, Canada

Introduction

Angiotensin-converting enzyme inhibitors (ACEI) employed in clinical practice for almost two decades, are now the most commonly prescribed class of cardiovascular agents. Indications for their use have grown substantially over this time period as information obtained through large clinical trials has enormously increased. Initially, captopril was prescribed in high doses for the treatment of hypertension until experience showed that lower doses of all ACEI were more effective. Eventually, they became an essential part of the therapeutic regimen against congestive heart failure and post-myocardial infarction. Our knowledge has also grown significantly to include their possible use in the prevention of diabetes with its micro- and macrovascular complications. They have also been administered successfully in patients with advanced renal failure of all etiologies.

More than ten different ACEI with greatly varying pharmacokinetic profiles are currently available on the market (Tab. 1). Although not all of them have been proven effective in modifying clinical outcomes in every situation, it is widely accepted that their benefits are due to class actions, proven by the use of specific agents. However, a debate is ongoing as to whether the beneficial consequences of ACEI should be considered class effects. In this review of the evidence underlying ACEI treatment of certain diseases, we will indicate the agents employed but will not discuss individual *versus* class effects.

In this chapter, we will summarize ACEI clinical trials assessing mortality and morbidity in hypertension, heart failure, myocardial infarction (MI), diabetes and renal failure. We also include studies on the effect of ACEI in patients with left ventricular hypertrophy (LVH), renal failure and diabetic retinopathy, as we consider these surrogate endpoints to be clinically important. Since the literature on the subject is extensive and thousands of clinical articles have been written concerning ACE inhibition in clinical settings, we have chosen only landmark trials that have governed the contemporary use of ACEI and that support current guidelines.

Table 1. Angiotensin converting enzyme inhibitors (ACEI), a comparative table

	Bénazépril	Captopril	Cilazapril	Énalapril	Fosinopril	Lisinopril	Périndopril	Quinapril	Ramipril
Indications									
Manufacturer	Novartis	Bristol Myers Squibb	Hoffman La Roche	Merck Frosst	Bristol Myers Squibb	Merck Frost Zénéca Ph	Servier	Pfizer	Aventis
Trademark	Lotensin	Capoten	Inhibace	Vasotec	Monopril	Prinivil/Zestril	Coversyl	Accupril	Altace
Hypertension	Mild to moderate hypertension	YES	Mild to moderate hypertension	YES	YES	YES	Mild to moderate hypertension	YES	YES
Heart failure	YES	YES	YES	YES	YES	YES	YES	YES	YES post MI
Dosage									
Usual initial dosage	5–10 mg	6.25–25 mg	0.5–2.5 mg	1.25–5 mg	5–10 mg	2.5–10 mg	2–4 mg	2.5–10 mg	1.25–5 mg
Usual dosage range	5–40 mg per day in 1 or 2 doses	12.5–150 mg per day in 2 or 3 doses	0.5–5 mg per day in 1 or 2 doses	1.25–20 mg per day in 1 or 2 doses	5–20 mg per day in 1 or 2 doses	2.5–40 mg per day in 1 dose	2–4 mg per day in 1 or 2 doses	2–20 mg per day in 1 or 2 doses	1.25–10 mg per day in 1 or 2 doses
maximum dosage	40 mg	150 mg	10 mg	40 mg	40 mg	80 mg	8 mg	40 mg	20 mg
Diuretics					Synergy				
Characteristics									
Lithium					Monitor serum concentration of lithium				
Main elimination route	Renal	Renal	Renal	Renal	Ren. 50%, Hep. 50% (may be adjusted)	Renal	Renal	Ren. 40%, Hep 60%	Ren. 40%, Hep 60%

Reproduced with permission from The Therapeutic Guide by the Société québécoise d'hypertension artérielle. March 1999: p 120–121

Hypertension

It was reported in the Framingham cohort study that hypertension is a major cardiovascular risk factor and that the risk of cardiovascular outcomes is linked to the level of systolic as well as diastolic blood pressure (BP) [1]. The Framingham study also reported on the additive effects of hypertension and other factors, such as cholesterol levels, blood glucose, cigarette smoking and LVH, on cardiovascular mortality and morbidity. The results of such epidemiological surveys led to intervention trials using various antihypertensive agents. The meta-analysis of MacMahon et al. [2, 3] showed that diastolic BP levels correlated directly with the prevalence of stroke and coronary heart disease (CHD). The higher the BP, the greater the incidence of stroke or CHD, which rises in a linear fashion from the diastolic BP level of 75 mmHg. A second meta-analysis of large intervention trials done worldwide until 1990 indicated that lowering BP with a beta-blocker or thiazide diuretic-based treatment is associated with a decreased incidence of stroke and cardiovascular events [3a]. The percentage reduction in stroke reported in these intervention trials was similar to the decline predicted from epidemiological studies. However, the percent diminution of coronary artery disease was significantly lower than the decrease predicted from epidemiological studies.

Non-diuretic or beta-blocker-based treatment regimens have also been associated with a fall in stroke and cardiovascular disease [4–7], but the evidence is not as strong. Accordingly, beta-blockers and thiazide diuretics have been recommended by some organizations (Joint National Committee, British Hypertension Society, Canadian Hypertension Society (JNC, BHS, CHS)) as initial therapy based on experience with these agents and the amount of available proof [8–10]. However, other groups such as the World Health Organization/International Society of Hypertension [11] recommend that since the prime link to the reduction of cardiovascular endpoints is the level of diastolic or systolic BP and since all trials used more than one agent, all forms of therapy that reduce BP can be given as initial treatment in hypertension as long as they are effective. A number of explanations have been advanced for this discrepancy: among them, the BP level obtained in the trials, the duration of treatment observation, the treatment of a single risk factor, and the type of antihypertensive agents used.

The target level of diastolic BP is a matter of debate. In large intervention trials on the benefit of antihypertensive agents, there were a significant number of participants who did not reach the target BP level of 90 mmHg: up to 30% in some centres. The Hypertension Optimal Treatment (HOT) trial [12] has addressed this question and reported that a diastolic BP of 82.6 mmHg was associated with the lowest incidence of major cardiovascular events, but there were no statistically significant differences within three groups of subjects whose diastolic BP was below 90 mmHg. In diabetics, reduction of BP to less than 80 mmHg was associated with a significant decrease in cardiovascular events.

Table 2. ACEI trials and hypertension

Study	Average or median age	Baseline blood pressure (mmHg)	Target treatment	Average follow up duration	Primary outcome	Results
CAPPP (1999) (N = 10,985)	53	160/99	Diastolic blood pressure less than 90 mmHg, captopril 50–100 mg daily vs conventionnal treatment	6.1 years	Fatal and non fatal myocardial infarction, stroke and cardiovascular death	No difference in myocardial infarctions and cardiovascular mortality but increase in stroke risk in captopril group
STOP-2 (1999) cardiovascular (N = 6614)	76	194/98	ACEI vs CCB vs older (Bblockers, diuretics) for target blood pressure less than 160/95	5 years	Cardiovascular mortality	No difference in mortality

All initial trials except HOT were conducted with a diuretic- or beta-blocker-based regimen. ACEI trials assessing clinical outcomes were only started recently. The Captopril Prevention Trial (CAPPP) (Tab. 2) reported by Hansson et al. [13] recently compared captopril to conventional therapy (beta-blockers and diuretics). Treatments did not differ in efficacy for the primary outcome (composite of fatal and non-fatal MI, stroke and other cardiovascular deaths). The same conclusion applied to individual cardiovascular outcomes except for stroke, which was more frequent in the captopril group (RR 1.25 CI: 1.01–1.55) and diabetes onset incidence, which was less frequent in the same group (RR 0.79 CI: 0.67–0.94). The difference in stroke risk could be explained by a small difference in baseline BP of 2 mmHg and the time period necessary to achieve the target BP, both favoring conventional treatment. In the subgroup of diabetics, the results very clearly favored ACEI over conventional treatment with fewer events. These findings suggest that ACEI are at least as effective as conventional therapy in a general population, and more effective in diabetic populations. The STOP-Hypertension-2 Study (Tab. 2) confirmed the equivalence of ACEI and conventional therapy (beta-blockers and diuretics) and showed an equal risk of stroke in both groups [14]. The only other trial on outcomes where ACEI were compared to conventional therapy was the UK Prospective Diabetes Study (UKPDS) which will be discussed in the Diabetes section.

ACE inhibitors are therefore antihypertensives that can be considered as initial therapy for uncomplicated hypertension based on the results of the CAPPP trial, the STOP-Hypertension-2 study, and also on the clearly established relationship between diastolic BP and cardiovascular events. The lower the BP, the greater the reduction of events with all tested agents. The question which is still unanswered is whether there is an added benefit to lowering BP by blocking angiotensin II synthesis than by another mechanism. A number of hypertension trials are in progress with ACEI [15, 16]. These trials are designed to compare the efficacy of different antihypertensive agents in reducing clinical outcomes. They are summarized in Table 11. ACEI are considered initial therapy or preferred therapy for hypertension and special conditions such as heart failure and diabetes which will be discussed in the following paragraphs.

Heart failure

Since the beginning of this decade, ACEI have become an accepted and strongly recommended treatment modality for patients with chronic congestive heart failure. At present these drugs are preferred for patients with symptomatic and asymptomatic systolic dysfunction by the American College of Cardiology and the American Heart Association [17, 18]. This practice is based on the results of large randomized clinical trials which examined the benefits of treating heart failure with ACEI *versus* other therapies. These studies on the use of ACEI in heart failure are summarized in Table 3 [19–23]. This list excludes tri-

Table 3. ACEI trials in heart failure (HF)

Study	Average or median age of patients	% of ischaemic heart failure	Ejection fraction (%)	Severity of HF	Treatment target	Average duration of follow up	Primary outcome	Results	NNT
CONSENSUS (1987) (N = 257)	71	57	NA	NYHA 4	Enalapril 10 mg bid vs placebo	188 days	Mortality at 6 months	Reduction in mortality (26 vs 44%) and improvement in NYHA classification in the enalapril group	6
SOLVD prevention (1991) (N = 2569)	59	83	28	Asympt.	Enalapril 10 mg bid vs placebo	37.4 months	Overall mortality	Non significant reduction in mortality but significant difference for combined outcomes (death and hospitalization)	
VHeFT II (1991) (N = 804)	61	53	29	NYHA 2-3	Enalapril 20 mg daily vs hydralazine 300 mg and isosorbide dinitrate 160 mg daily	2.5 years	Mortality at 2 years	Reduction in mortality at 2 years (18 vs 25%) and trend in reducing overall mortality in the enalapril group	14
SOLVD Treatment (1992) (N = 4228)	61	71	25	NYHA 2-3	Enalapril vs placebo	41.4 months	Overall mortality	Reduction in overall mortality in the enalapril group (35.2 vs 39.7%)	22
ELITE (1997) (N = 722)	74	68	30	NYHA 2-4	Losartan 50 mg die vs Captopril 50 mg tid	48 weeks	Creatinine elevation at 48 weeks	No difference in primary outcome but an unexpected lower mortality in the Losartan group (4.8 vs 8.7%)	26

NNT: number needed to treat for one life saved

als of post acute MI. The combined results strongly indicate that enalapril reduces total mortality in patients with heart failure. From these studies, we can also conclude that symptomatic patients benefit more than asymptomatic patients [22]. The equivalence of high-dose vs low-dose of ACEI and ACEI vs AT2 blockers is, however, still being debated. In the ATLAS trial [24] where 3,164 patients with moderate to severe heart failure were randomized to low-dose or high-dose lisinopril, high doses were superior to low doses in decreasing the combined risk of death or hospitalization (79.8 vs 83.9%) and were generally as well tolerated as low doses. In the Evaluation of Losartan in the Elderly Study (ELITE) [23] designed to investigate renal failure, 722 elderly ACEI naive patients with heart failure (NYHA 2-4) were randomized to losartan 50 mg daily or captopril 50 mg t.i.d. There was no significant difference in primary outcome, but a surprising statistically significant reduction in total mortality was observed in favor of losartan. Preliminary results of ELITE II study, designed to evaluate all causes mortality of losartan compared to captopril, have indicated, however, that there was no statistically significant difference in all causes mortality or in sudden cardiac death [25].

It is therefore clear that high-dose ACEI is more beneficial than low-dose ACEI. If not tolerated, AT1 receptor blockers, such as losartan, are acceptable and probably an equivalent alternative. Preliminary results from the Valsartan Heart Failure Trial (Val-Heft) suggest that the beneficial effects of ACEI and AT1 receptor blockers are not additive. Their combination cannot be recommended at this point in time.

Post-MI heart failure

Post-MI heart failure has a different clinical presentation than chronic heart failure. Frequently associated with recent cardiopulmonary instability, physicians were reticent to prescribe what was perceived as being an antihypertensive agent to a non hypertensive patient. Before 1992, laboratory data had shown beneficial effects of chronic ACEI treatment on ventricular remodeling [26, 27] but clinical trials were needed. The Survival and Ventricular Enlargement (SAVE) trial was the first to demonstrate convincingly that 42 months of treatment with captopril reduced mortality and cardiovascular events in post-MI heart failure [28]. The results were the same if the patients had or had not received thrombolytics, aspirin or beta-blockers. Since then, two clinical trials, one comparing trandolapril to placebo (TRACE) [29], and the other comparing ramipril to placebo (AIRE) [30, 31], in patients with transient or ongoing heart failure after MI, have confirmed these data. See Table 4 for a summary of post-MI heart failure trials.

At present, ACEI are recommended by the American College of Cardiology and the American Heart Association for all patients with post-MI heart failure [18].

Table 4. ACEI trials in post myocardial infarction heart failure

Study	Average or median age of patients	Ejection fraction (%)	Treatment target	Time after MI (mean days)	Average duration of follow up	Primary outcome	Results	NNT
SAVE (1992) (N = 2231)	59	31	Captopril 25 mg tid vs placebo	11	42 months	Overall mortality	Reduction in overall mortality in the captopril group (20 vs 25%) and reduced morbidity	20
AIRE (1993) (N = 2006)	65	NA	Ramipril 5 mg bid vs placebo	5.4	15 months	Overall mortality	Reduction in overall mortality (17 vs 23%) and reduction of cardio-vascular events in the ramipril group	17
TRACE (1995) (N = 1749)	67	<35	Trandolapril 4 mg die	4.5	NA but ranges from 24 to 50 months (599 patients left at 36 months and 42 at 48 months)	Overall mortality	Reduction in overall mortality (34.7 vs 42.3%) and reduced progression to severe heart failure in the trandolapril group	13
AIREX (1997) (N = 603)	65	44	Ramipril 5 mg bid for an average of placebo 12.4 months vs placebo for an average of 13.4 months	5.04	59 months	Overall mortality	Reduction in overall mortality (27.5 vs 38.9%)	11

NA: not available, NNT: number needed to treat for one life saved

Acute MI

Treatment of MI always has the objective of increasing the ratio between oxygen delivery and consumption. During acute MI, the sympathetic and renin-angiotensin systems are activated and are believed to be instrumental in the ventricular remodeling process [32]. Different treatment modalities counteracting these reflex mechanisms have been investigated. Promising animal as well as human studies have led to the design of the CONSENSUS II trial comparing enalapril to placebo in acute MI [33]. Surprisingly, a trend of increasing mortality with ACEI forced early termination of the trial and stirred debate on the causes of such results. This uncertainty led to the design of the GISSI-3 trial, a wide multicenter, factorial, placebo-controlled clinical study assessing the effects of a six-week treatment with lisinopril and transdermal glyceryl trinitrate in acute MI [34]. The results showed a statistically significant reduction in mortality alone or combined with heart failure. Since then, other trials using different ACEI have confirmed the GISSI-3 data [35–40]. They are summarized in Table 5.

Recommendations for the treatment of acute MI were revised in 1999 by the American Heart Association [41] and reiterated 1996 guidelines. ACEI should be used within 24 h of MI if systolic BP is over 100 mmHg, and if no contraindications to ACEI are present.

Diabetes

Diabetes is widely prevalent and is a major cardiovascular disease risk factor. Strict BP control and the use of ACEI for diabetic nephropathy have been strongly emphasized in past years [8–11, 42, 43]. Table 6 summarizes studies involving ACEI in diabetic hypertensive patients [44–46]. The UKPDS trial comparing captopril and atenolol in hypertensive diabetic subjects [46] did not report differences in BP reduction, death and diabetes-related clinical endpoints. The FACET and ABCD trials [44, 45], both comparing ACEI with calcium channel blockers, found a decrease in cardiovascular and death outcomes in the ACEI group. It is noteworthy that both these trials had primary outcomes that were unrelated to cardiovascular mortality or morbidity. Therefore, the UKPDS study should be considered the most reliable reference on this subject. ACEI and beta-blockers should be made the first-line antihypertensive treatment in diabetic hypertensive subjects.

Glomerular pressure having been implicated in deterioration of renal function, ACEI have long been considered possible renoprotective agents. Diabetes has been studied specifically as the most common cause of chronic renal failure. Animal and small clinical trials suggested that ACEI preserved renal function [46–50]. Major trials primarily assessing renal function in normotensive diabetic patients were, therefore, designed and are summarized in Table 7 [51–54]. Lewis et al. [51] and the EUCLID Study Group [52] analyzed the use

Table 5. ACEI trials in acute myocardial infarction

Study	Average or median age of patients	Killip class (%)	Treatment target	Time after MI (mean days)	Duration of tratment	Average duration of follow up	Primary outcome	Results	NNT
CONSENSUS II (1992) (N = 6090)	66	11% had hypotension and 3% had pulmonary oedema	Enalaprilat IV followed by enalapril 20 mg daily vs placebo	<24 h	6 months	NA but when trial was stopped, 2952 had been followed for 180 days	Mortality at 6 months	Stopped early trend in increasing mortality in the enalapril group (11 vs 10.2%)	
GISSI-3 (1994) (N = 19394)	NA but 27% > 70 years	1–85%, 2–14%, 3–1%	Lisinopril 10 mg daily vs open conrol	<24 h	6 weeks	NA but 97.4% of subjects completed 6 weeks of follow up	Mortality at 6 weeks	Reduction in mortality (6.3 vs 7.1%) and combined death and severe heart failure in the lisinopril group	125
SMILE (1995) (N = 1556)	64	1–86%, >1–14%	Zofenopril 30 mg bid vs placebo	<24 h	6 weeks	NA but 100% of patients are used for 6 weeks and 12 months results	Mortality at 6 weeks	Reduction in combined mortality and severe heart failure (7.1 vs 10.6%) in the zofenopril group and survival advantage was maintained at 12 months	
ISIS-4 (1995) (N = 58040)	NA but 28% >70 years	NA	Captopril 50 mg bid vs placebo	<24 h	1 month	NA but 97% of follow up at 5 weeks and 68% at 12 months	Mortality at 5 weeks	Reduction in mortality in the captopril group (7.19 vs 7.69%) and survival advantage maintained at 12 months	200
CCS1 (1997) (N = 14962)	NA	NA	Captopril 12.5 mg tid vs placebo	<36 h	4 weeks	NA but 90% of subjects completed the 4 weeks study period	Mortality at 4 weeks	Non significant reduction in mortality (9.12 vs 10.7% but reduction of heart failure (21.5 vs 23.1%)	

(continued on next page)

Table 5. (continued)

Study	Average or median age of patients	Killip class (%)	Treatment target	Time after MI (mean days)	Duration of tratment	Average duration of follow up	Primary outcome	Results	NNT
FAMIS (1998) (N = 285)	60	1–80%, >1–20	Fosinopril 20 mg daily vs placebo	<9 h	3 months	24 months	Left ventricular volume at 3 months	No difference for primary outcome but reduction in the 2 year combined mortality and heart failure rates (17.5 vs 26.8%)	
CATS (1994) (N = 298)	60	1–75%, 2–25%	Captopril 25 mg tid vs placebo	<6 h		NA but 94.6% of subjects completed 3 months follow-up	Left ventricular volume at 3 months	No difference for primary outcome but reduction in the incidence of heart failure in the captopril group (18.7 vs 28.2)	

NA: not available, NNT: number needed to treat for one life saved

Table 6. ACEI trials in diabetic hypertensive patients

Study	Average or median age of patients	Type of diabetes	Treatment target	Average duration of follow up	Primary outcome(s)	Results
FACET (1998) (N = 380)	63	2	Fosinopril 20 mg daily vs amlodipine 10 mg daily	2.5 years	Blood pressure reduction, serum lipids and diabetes control	No difference for primary outcomes but lower risk for combined acute MI, stroke or hospitalization for angina in the fosinopril group (7.4 vs 14.1%)
ABCD (1998) (N = 470)	57	2	Enalapril 40 mg daily vs nisoldipine 60 mg daily	NA but survival curves extend to 60 months	Creatinine clearance	Termination of trial for hypertensive patients. Lower incidence of MI in the enalapril group (2.1% vs 10.6%)
UKPDS 39 (1998) (N = 758)	56	2	Captopril 50 mg bid vs atenolol 100 mg daily	NA but 644 subjects completed follow up at 3 years, 493 at 6 years and 235 at 9 years	Death from all causes, death related to diabetes and first clinical end-point related to diabetes	No difference for primary outcomes and no difference in deterioration of retinopathy

Table 7. ACEI trials in diabetic non-hypertensive patients

Study	Average or median age of patients	Mean baseline blood pressure (mmHg)	Type of diabetes	Proteinuria	Treatment target days)	Average duration of follow up	Primary outcome(s)	Results
Lewis et al. (1993) (N = 409)	35	103	1	All had proteinuria >500 mg/day	Captopril 25 mg tid vs placebo	1.7 years	Doubling of the base-line creatinine concentration	Lower incidence of the primary endpoint in the captopril group (12.0 vs 21.2%)
EUCLID (1997) (N = 530)	33	94	1	86% normoalbuminuria, 13% microalbuminuria, 1% macroalbuminuria	Lisinopril 20 mg daily vs placebo	NA but 465 subjects attended final visit at 2 years	Microalbuminuria evolution at 2 years	Lower albumin excretion rate in the lisinopril group (2.2 ug/min) with greater benefits in the microalbuminuric group
EUCLID (1998) (N = 409)	35	95	1		Lisinopril 20 mg daily vs placebo	NA but 354 subjects attended final visit at 2 years	Retinopathy evolution at 2 years	Lisinopril may decrease retinopathy progression
Ravid et al. (1998) (N = 194)	55	97	2	normoalbuminuria	Enalapril 10 mg daily vs placebo	NA but 156 subjects completed the protocol	Microalbuminuria at 6 years	Enalapril decreased microalbuminuria progression and attenuated clearance decrease

NA: not available

of ACEI in type I diabetes while Ravid et al. [53] focused on type 2 diabetes. The combined results of these trials strongly suggest that ACEI have renoprotective properties in normotensive diabetic patients. Subjects with microalbuminuria (30–300 mg/24 h) or overt proteinuria (>300 mg/24 h) should probably expect more benefits than normoalbuminuric patients. The EUCLID Study Group also analyzed the relationship between ACE gene polymorphism, albumin excretion rate (AER) progression and the response to lisinopril. They found that certain alleles (II) of the ACE gene were related to increased AER progression on placebo but manifested an enhanced response to lisinopril [55].

Diabetic retinopathy is the most frequent cause of blindness in North America, and tight glycemic control remains the main intervention that prevents its development and slows its progression. Even if hypertension is a well-known risk factor for retinopathy, it is not certain if antihypertensive agents can have beneficial effects in diabetic retinopathy. Two trials addressed this issue. The UKPDS trial [46] found a similar proportion of patients with deterioration in retinopathy in the captopril and atenolol groups and the EUCLID Study Group [54] observed a decrease in retinopathy progression when lisinopril was compared to placebo. Neither of these studies was designed with retinopathy as a primary outcome. More trials will be needed to confirm these results.

There were fewer new cases of diabetes in the CAPPP and Heart Outcomes Prevention Evaluation (HOPE) studies than with conventional control treatment. This preventive result will have to be defined more clearly in ongoing trials evaluating different forms of treatment, such as the ALLHAT study (Tab. 11) [15].

At present, recommendations state that ACEI should be used in type 1 and 2 diabetic patients who have microalbuminuria (30–300 mg/24 h) or overt proteinuria (>300 mg/24 h) [43] whether they are hypertensive or normotensive. Guidelines differ in their recommendation of the ideal antihypertensive in diabetic patients without nephropathy or microalbuminuria, but all include ACEI [8–11, 43]. In such cases, the strongest evidence comes from the UKPDS-39 [46] study and supports the use of beta-blockers or ACEI as initial therapy.

Left ventricular hypertrophy

LVH is a well-known and strong marker of cardiovascular morbidity and mortality in patients with hypertension [56]. In itself, LVH carries a risk of diastolic heart failure and an increase in ventricular arrhythmias [57]. It has been suggested that reversing hypertension-related structural cardiovascular changes such as LVH may be a more important objective than lowering BP [57–59]. It is still unknown though if LVH reduction can cut cardiovascular risk independently of BP. There is also no definite prospective evidence that LVH reversal diminishes cardiovascular risk. It is debateable whether some antihypertensive drugs are more effective than others in decreasing left ventricular mass (LVM) independently of BP reduction. Three well-known meta-analyses by Dahlöf [60], Schmieder et al. [61] and Jennings and Wong [62], differ in their conclusions. In the first two, ACEI seem to be clearly more effective than other antihypertensives in reducing LVH, but in the latter, ACEI were second to calcium channel blockers and not more effective than other antihypertensives. Beta-blockers were the only antihypertensives that consistently had a smaller effect on LVH in the three meta-analyses. From the prospective trials summarized in Table 8 [63–66], we can only conclude that ACEI decrease LVM more effectively than placebo, and it is still unclear if they are more or less effective than other antihypertensives. The RACE trial [65] seems to show greater LVM reduction with ACEI in comparison to beta-blockers, but this action does not appear in TOMHS [63].

From the available evidence, ACEI seem to be at least equivalent or superior to other antihypertensives in reducing LVH, with the exception of beta-blockers that seem to be less effective in most studies.

One ACEI LVH (PRESERVE) trial is in progress and is designed to compare the effects of enalapril vs nifedipine in reducing LVH [67]. It is summarized in Table 11.

Non-diabetic renal failure

Recently, in a review of the literature on renoprotection, Burgess [68] proposed some recommendations on the use of ACEI in hypertensive patients suffering from non-diabetic renal failure. It was stated that ACEI are preferable to placebo or beta-blockers when treating renal disease but the evidence suggests that there is no difference between the long term renoprotection of ACEI and CCBs. Meta-analysis by Giatras et al. [69] has shown greater renoprotection associated with ACEI but cannot distinguish a possible class effect from the lower BPs that were attained.

From the main ACEI trials on renal failure summarized in Table 9 [70–74], it appears that ACEI have better renoprotective properties than conventional treatment or beta-blockers in non-diabetic patients. There might be a trend favoring ACEI over calcium channel blockers, but not enough evidence supports this hypothesis. It also appears that normotensive or mildly hypertensive patients suffering from renal failure can benefit from ACEI.

High risk patients

The concept is growing that ACEI could prevent cardiovascular morbidity and death in subjects at high risk of cardiovascular events who do not suffer from heart failure or acute MI. Ongoing clinical trials are addressing this subject, and results should be available in the near future [75–79]. Table 10 summarizes the recently published HOPE study [80]. Stopped early, it showed an

Table 8. ACEI trials and left ventricular hypertrophy

Study	Average or median age of patients	Treatment target	Average duration of follow up	Primary outcome	Results
TOMHS (1995) (N = 844)	55	Enalapril 5 mg daily vs chlorthalidone 15 mg daily vs Acebutolol 400 mg daily vs doxasozin 2 mg daily vs amlodipine 5 mg daily vs placebo	NA but 718 subjects completed protocol at 12 months	Left ventricular mass	Trend towards having lower left ventricular mass in the active group at 12 months (-23.6 vs -18.2 g) but not at 4 years. chlorthalidone was the most beneficial (-34.8 g at 12 months)
Gottdiener et al. (1997) (N = 1105)	58	Captopril vs atenolol vs clonidine vs diltiazem vs hydrochlorothiazide vs prazosin for diastolic blood pressure of <90 mmHg	NA but 493 subjects completed protocol at 1 year	Left ventricular mass	Patients with adequate blood pressure control on captopril (-38.7 g), hydrochlorothiazide (-42.9 g) and atenolol (-28.1 g) had reduced left ventricular mass compared to clonidine (-0.5 g), diltiazem (-6.9 g) and prazosin (-5.9 g)
HYCAR (1995) (N = 115)	53	Ramipril 5 mg daily vs ramipril 1.25 mg daily vs placebo	6 months	Left ventricular mass	Ramipril 5 mg had lower left ventricular mass compared to placebo (-10.8 vs $+4.1$ g/m^2) and ramipril 1.25 mg had a non significant lower left ventricular mass compared with placebo
RACE (1995) (N = 111)		Ramipril vs atenolol	6 months	Left ventricular mass	Ramipril had lower left ventricular mass compared to atenolol

NA: not available

Table 9. ACEI trials in renal failure

Study	Average or median age	Percent of diabetes	Baseline average blood pressure (mmHg)	Average proteinuria	Target treatment	Average duration of follow up	Primary outcome	Results
Zuchelli et al. (1992) (N = 121)	55	0	144	1.78 g/24 h.	Captopril 50 mg bid vs Nifédipine 20 mg bid	NA but 69 patients completed the 3 year protocol	Need for dialysis	Non significant decrease in primary outcome in the captopril group at 3 years
Hannedouche et al. (1994) (N = 100)	51	0	124	2.2 g/24 h	Enalapril vs β blocker for diastolic blood pressure <90 mmHg	NA but 52 subjects completed the 3 year protocol	End-stage renal failure	Reduced primary outcome at 3 years (19 vs 35%) and reduced proteinuria in the enalapril group
Maschio et al. (1996) (N = 583)	51	3%	106	1.8 g/24 h	Benazepril 10 mg daily vs placebo	NA but 428 subjects completed the 2 year protocol and 135 completed the 3 year protocol	Doubling of the base-line serum creatinine	Less patients reached the primary end point in the benazepril group at 3 years (10.3 vs 20.1%)
REIN (1997) (N = 166)	49	0	111	5.3 g/24 h	Ramipril for diastolic blood pressure <90 mmHg vs placebo	16 months	Rate of decline of the GFR	Decline in GFR (0.53 vs 0.88 cc/min) and proteinuria were lower in the ramipril group

GFR: glomerular filtration rate

Table 10. ACEI trials in high risk patients without heart failure

Study	Average or median age of patients	Inclusion criteria	Treatment target	Average duration of follow up	Primary outcome	Results	NNT
HOPE (2000) (N = 9297)	66	High risk for cardiovascular events (any evidence of vascular disease or diabetes + other risk factor). Heart failure excluded	Ramipril 10 mg daily vs placebo	4–6 years intended cardiovascular death	Combined: heart attack, stroke and	Ended prematurely. Reduction of the primary outcome (13.9 vs 17.5%), reduction in mortality (10.6 vs 13.9%)	30

NNT: number needed to treat for one life saved

Table 11. ACEI trials in progress

Study	Expected average age	Study population	Treatment targets	Expected follow up	Primary outcome
Elite II (N = 3152)	72	Subjects with heart failure and EF < 40%	Losartan 50 mg daily vs captopril 50 mg tid	Until 510 events occur	Overall mortality
PRESERVE (N = 480)	>50	Non hypertensive with high left ventricular mass	Enalapril 20 mg daily vs nifédipine 60 mg daily	12 months	Left ventricular mass and diastolic filling
PEACE (N = 8100)	>50	Patients with CHD and no heart failure	trandolapril 4 mg daily vs placebo	5.5 years	Cardiovascular mortality and morbidity
EUROPA (N = 10,500)	>18	Patients with CHD and no heart failure	Perindopril	3.5 years	Mortality and cardiac events
DIAB-HYCAR (N = 4000)	>50	NIDDM with persistent microalbuminuria	1.25 mg ramipril vs placebo	3 years	Cardiovascular mortality and morbidity
PROGRESS (N = 6000)	NA	CVA or TIA in the past 5 years	perindopril 4 mg plus indapamide 2.5 mg daily vs placebo	4 years	Stroke
ALLHAT (N = 40,000)	>55 years	High risk hypertensive patients	diuretic plus amlodipine or lisinopril or doxazosin	6 years	Fatal and non fatal CHD
ANBP2 (N = 6000)	65–84	Hypertension	ACEI vs diuretic based treatment	5 years	Fatal and non fatal cardiovascular events

NA: not available

absolute reduction of 3.6% (13.9% vs 17.5%) in combined heart attack, stroke and cardiovascular death outcomes. Obviously, a study of such clinical importance needs to be further analyzed and peer reviewed, but it seems likely that ACEI use in high risk patients will become part of clinical practice.

Conclusion

In conclusion, we would like to underscore that no other drug class in the past 20 years has had more impact on cardiovascular disease than ACEI. Justifiably, ACEI are considered safe, potent and life-saving drugs in heart failure, MI, hypertension and diabetes. New and promising virtues of ACEI are being studied, and we believe an increase in ACEI use is to be expected in the near future. Some are already evaluating the cost-effectiveness of ACEI in primary prevention [81] but we cannot advocate such a practice at this time because ACEI are not devoid of adverse effects. We can be optimistic though that future clinical trial results and genotyping will identify population subgroups that may benefit from earlier treatment with ACEI.

Acknowledgements
The authors wish to thank Lise Lussier for her clerical support and Ovid Da Silva for editing the manuscript.

References

1 Kannel WB, McGee D, Gordon T (1976) A general cardiovascular risk profile: The Framingham Study. *Amer J Cardiol* 38: 46–51
2 MacMahon S, Peto R, Cutler J, Collins R, Sorlie P, Neaton J, Abbott R, Godwin J, Dyer A, Stamler J (1990) Blood pressure, stroke, and coronary heart disease. Part 1. Prolonged differences in blood pressure: Prospective observational studies corrected for the regression dilution bias. *Lancet* 335: 765–774
3 Collins R, Peto R, MacMahon S, Hebert P, Fiebach NH, Eberlein KA, Godwin J, Qizilbash N, Taylor JO, Hennekens CH (1990) Blood pressure, stroke, and coronary heart disease. Part 2. Short-term reductions in blood pressure: Overview of randomised drug trials in their epidemiological context. *Lancet* 335: 827–838
3a Gueyffier F, Boutitie F, Boissel JP, Pocock S, Coope J, Cutler J, Ekbom T, Fagard R, Friedmann L, Perry M et al (1997) Effect of antihypertensive drug treatment on cardiovascular outcomes in women and men. A meta-analysis of individual patient data from randomized, controlled trials. The INDANA Investigators. *Ann Intern Med* 126: 761–767
4 Staessen JA, Fagard R, Thijs L, Celis H, Arabidze GG, Birkenhäger WH, Bulpitt CJ, deLeeuw PW, Dollery CT, Fletcher AE et al (1997) Randomised double-blind comparison of placebo and active treatment for older patients with isolated systolic hypertension. *Lancet* 350: 757–764
5 Liu L, Wang JG, Gong L, Liu G, Staessen JA (1998) Comparison of active treatment and placebo in older Chinese patients with isolated systolic hypertension. Systolic Hypertension in China (Syst-China) Collaborative Group. *J Hypertension* 16 (12 Pt 1): 1823–1829
6 Hansson L (1999) The Hypertension Optimal Treatment study and the importance of lowering blood pressure. *J Hypertension* 17 (1) S9–S13
7 Gong L, Zhang W, Zhu Y, Zhu J, 11 collaborating centres in the Shanghai area Kong D, Pagé V, Ghadirian P, Le Lorier J, Hamet P (1996) Shanghai trial of nifedipine in the elderly (STONE). *J*

Hypertension 14: 1237–1245

8   The Sixth Report of the Joint National Committee on Prevention Detection Evaluation, Treatment of High Blood Pressure (1997) NIH Publication No. 98–4080

9   Ramsay LE, Williams B, Johnston GD, MacGregor GA, Poston L, Potter JF, Poulter NR, Russel G (1999) British Hypertension Society guidelines for hypertension management 1999: summary. *BMJ* 319: 630–635

10 Feldman RD, Campbell N, Larochelle P, Bolli P, Burgess ED, Carruthers SG, Floras JS, Haynes RB, Honos G, Leenen FHH (1999) Recommandations de 1999 pour le traitement de l'hypertension artérielle au Canada. *CMAJ* 161 (suppl 12): SF1–SF25

11 Guidelines Subcommittee (WHO –ISH) (1999) World Health Organization – International Society of Hypertension Guidelines for the Management of Hypertension. *J Hypertension* 17: 151–183

12 Hansson L, Zanchetti A, Carruthers SG, Dahlöf B, Elmfeldt D, Julius S, Ménard J, Rahn KH, Wedel H, Westerling S for the HOT Study Group (1998) Effects of intensive blood pressure-lowering and low-dose aspirin in patients with hypertension: Principal results of the Hypertension Optimal Treatment (HOT) randomised trial. *Lancet* 351: 1755–1762

13 Hansson L, Lindholm LH, Niskanen L, Lanke J, Hedner T, Niklason A, Luomanmäki K, Dahlöf B, de Faire U, Mörlin C (1999) Effects of angiotensin-converting enzyme inhibition compared with conventional therapy on cardiovascular morbidity and mortality in hypertension. *Lancet* 353: 611–616

14 Hansson L, Lindholm LH, Ekbom T, Dahlöf B, Lanke J, Scherstén B, Wester PO, Hedner T, de Faire U for the STOP-Hypertension-2 Study Group (1999) Randomised trial of old and new antihypertensive drugs in elderly patients: Cardiovascular mortality and morbidity. The Swedish Trial in Old Patients with Hypertension-2 study. *Lancet* 354: 1751–1756

15 Davis BR, Cutler JA, Gordon DJ, Furberg CD, Wright JTJr Cushman WC, Grimm RH, LaRosa J, Whelton PK, Perry HM (1996) Rationale and design for the antihypertensive and lipid lowering treatment to prevent heart attack trial (ALLHAT). *Amer J Hypertens* 9 (4): 342–360

16 Management Committee on behalf of the High Blood Pressure Research Council of Australia (1997) Australian comparative outcome trial of angiotensin-converting enzyme inhibitor and diuretic based treatment of hypertension in the elderly (ANBP2): Objectives and protocol. *Clin Exp Pharmacol Physiol* 24 (2): 188–192

17 Consensus recommendations for the management of chronic heart failure (1999) *Amer J Cardiol* 83 (2A): 1A–38A

18 Report of the American College of Cardiology/American Heart Association Task Force on Practice Guidelines (Committee on Evaluation, Management of Heart Failure) (1995) Guidelines for the evaluation and Management of heart failure. *Circulation* 92: 2764–2784

19 The SOLVDInvestigators (1991) Effect of enalapril on survival in patients with reduced left ventricular ejection fractions and congestive heart failure. *N Engl J Med* 325: 293–302

20 Cohn JN, Johnson G, Ziesche S, Cobb F, Francis G, Tristani F, Smith R, Dunkman WB, Loeb H, Wong M (1991) A comparison of enalapril with hydralazine-isosorbide dinitrate in the treatment of chronic congestive heart failure. *N Engl J Med* 325 (5): 303–310

21 The Consensus Trial Study Group (1987) Effects of enalapril on mortality in severe congestive heart failure. Results of the Cooperative North Scandinavian Enalapril Survival Study (Consensus). *N Engl J Med* 316 (23): 1429–1435

22 The SOLVDInvestigators (1992) Effect of enalapril on mortality and the development of heart failure in asymptomatic patients with reduced left ventricular ejection fractions. *N Engl J Med* 327: 685–691

23 Pitt B, Segal R, Martinez FA, Meurers G, Cowley AJ, Thomas I, Deedwania PC, Ney DE, Snavely DB, Chang PI, on behalf of ELITEStudy Investigators (1997) Randomised trial of losartan *versus* captopril in patients over 65 with heart failure (Evaluation of Losartan in the Elderly Study, ELITE). *Lancet* 349: 747–752

24 Packer M, Poole-Wilson P, Armstrong P, Cleland J, Horowitz J, Massie B, Ryden L, Thygesen K, Uretsky BF (1999) Comparative effects of low and high doses of the angiotensin-converting enzyme inhibitor, lisinopril, on morbidity and mortality in chronic heart failure. ATLAS Study Group. *Circulation* 100 (23): 2312–2318

25 Pitt B, Poole-Wilson P, Segal R, Martinez FA, Dickstein K, Camm AJ, Konstam MA, Riegger G, Klinger GH, Neaton J (1999) Effects of losartan *versus* captopril on mortality in patients with symptomatic heart failure: Rationale, design, and baseline characteristics of patients in the losartan heart failure survival study – ELITE. *Cardiac Failure* 5 (2): 146–154

26 Pfeffer MA, Lamas GA, Vaughan DE, Parisi AF, Braunwald E (1988) Effect of captopril on progressive ventricular dilatation after anterior myocardial infarction. *N Engl J Med* 319: 80–86

27 Sharpe N, Murphy J, Smith H, Hannan S (1988) Treatment of patients with symptomless left ventricular dysfunction after myocardial infarction. *Lancet* 6: 255–259

28 Pfeffer MA, Braunwald E, Moyé LA, Basta L, Brown EJJr Cuddy TE, Davis BR, Geltman EM, Goldman S, Flaker GC (1992) Effect of captopril on mortality and morbidity in patients with left ventricular dysfunction after myocardial infarction. *N Engl J Med* 327: 669–679

29 Kober L, Torp-Pedersen C, Carlsen JE, Bagger H, Eliasen P, Lyngborg K, Videbaek J, Cole DS, Auclert L, Pauly NC (1995) A clinical trial of the angiotensin-converting enzyme inhibitor trandolapril in patients with left ventricular dysfunction after myocardial infarction. *N Engl J Med* 333: 1670–1676

30 The Acute Infarction Ramipril Efficacy (AIRE) Study Investigators (1993) Effect of ramipril on mortality and morbidity of survivors of acute myocardial infarction with clinical evidence of heart failure. *Lancet* 342: 821–828

31 Hall AS, Murray GD, Ball SG on behalf of the AIREXStudy Investigators (1997) Follow-up study of patients randomly allocated ramipril or placebo for heart failure after acute myocardial infarction: AIRE Extension (AIREX) Study. *Lancet* 349: 1493–1497

32 McAlpine HM, Morton JJ, Leckie B, Rumley A, Gillen G, Dargie HJ (1988) Neuroendocrine activation after acute myocardial infarction. *Brit Heart J* 60: 117–124

33 Swedberg K, Held P, Kjekshus J, Rasmussen K, Rydén L, Wedel H on behalf of the Consensus IIStudy Group (1992) Effects of the early administration of enalapril on mortality in patients with acute myocardial infarction. *N Engl J Med* 327: 678–684

34 Gruppo Italiano per lo Studio della Sopravvivenza nell'Infarto Miocardico (1994) GISSI-3: Effects of lisinopril and transdermal glyceryl trinitrate singly and together on 6-week mortality and ventricular function after acute myocardial infarction. *Lancet* 343: 1115–1122

35 Kingma JH, Van Gilst WH, Peels CH, Dambrink JHE, Verheugt FWA, Wielenga RP for the CATSInvestigators (1994) Acute intervention with captopril during thrombolysis in patients with first anterior myocardial infarction. *Eur Heart J* 15: 898–907

36 Ambrosioni E, Borghi C, Magnani B for the Survival of Myocardial Infarction Long-Term Evaluation (SMILE) Study Investigators (1995) The effect of the angiotensin-converting-enzyme inhibitor zofenopril on mortality and morbidity after anterior myocardial infarction. *N Engl J Med* 332: 80–85

37 ISIS-4 (Fourth International Study of Infarct Survival) Collaborative Group (1995) *Isis* 4: A randomised factorial trial assessing early oral captopril, oral mononitrate, and intravenous magnesium sulphate in 58,050 patients with suspected acute myocardial infarction. *Lancet* 345: 669–685

38 Chinese Cardiac Study Collaborative Group (1995) Oral captopril *versus* placebo among 13,634 patients with suspected acute myocardial infarction: Interim report from the Chinese Cardiac Study (CCS-1). *Lancet* 345: 686–687

39 Chinese Cardiac Study (CCS-1) Collaborative Group (1997) Oral captopril *versus* placebo among 14,962 patients with suspected acute myocardial infarction: A multicenter, randomized, double-blind placebo controlled clinical trial. *Chin Med J* 110 (11): 834–838

40 Borghi C, Marino P, Zardini P, Magnani B, Collatina S, Ambrosioni E for the FAMISWorking Party Bologna Verona, Rome Italy (1998) Short- and long-term effects of early fosinopril administration in patients with acute anterior myocardial infarction undergoing intravenous thrombolysis: Results from the Fosinopril in Acute Myocardial Infarction Study. *Amer Heart J* 136: 213–225

41 Report of the American College of Cardiology/American Heart Association Task Force on Practice Guidelines (Committee on Management of Acute Myocardial Infarction) (1996) ACC/AHA guidelines for the management of patients with acute myocardial infarction. *JACC* 28 (5): 1328–1428

42 Ritz E, Orth SR (1999) Nephropathy in patients with type 2 diabetes mellitus. *N Engl J Med* 341: 1127–1133

43 Meltzer S, Leiter L, Daneman D, Gerstein HC, Lau D, Ludwig S, Yale JF, Zinman B, Lillie D, Comité directeur et Comité d'experts (1998) Lignes directrices de pratique clinique 1998 pour le traitement du diabète au Canada. *CMAJ* 159 (suppl 8): S1–S31

44 Estacio RO, Jeffers BW, Hiatt WR, Biggerstaff SL, Gifford N, Schrier RW (1998) The effect of nisoldipine as compared with enalapril on cardiovascular outcomes in patients with non-insulin-dependent diabetes and hypertension. *N Engl J Med* 338: 645–652

45 Tatti P, Pahor M, Byington RP, Di Mauro P, Guarisco R, Strollo G, Strollo F (1998) Outcome

results of the fosinopril *versus* amlodipine cardiovascular events randomized trial (FACET) in patients with hypertension and NIDDM. *Diabetes Care* 21: 597–603

46 UKProspective Diabetes Study Group (1998) Efficacy of atenolol and captopril in reducing risk of macrovascular and microvascular complications in type 2 diabetes: UKPDS 39. *BMJ* 317: 713–720

47 Anderson S, Rennke HG, Garcia DL, Brenner BM with the technical assistance of Riley SL, Sandstrom DJ (1989) Short and long-term effects of antihypertensive therapy in the diabetic rat. *Kidney Int* 36: 526–536

48 Hommel E, Parving HH, Mathiesen E, Edsberg B, Nielsen MD, Giese J (1986) Effect of captopril on kidney function in insulin-dependent diabetic patients with nephropathy. *BMJ* 293: 467–470

49 Parving HH, Hommel E, Smidt UM (1988) Protection of kidney function and decrease in albuminuria by captopril in insulin dependent diabetics with nephropathy. *BMJ* 297: 1086–1091

50 Marre M, Chatellier G, Leblanc H, Guyene TT, Menard J, Passa P (1988) Prevention of diabetic nephropathy with enalapril in normotensive diabetics with microalbuminuria. *BMJ* 297: 1092–1095

51 Lewis EJ, Hunsicker LG, Bain RP, Rohde RD for the Collaborative Study Group (1993) The effect of angiotensin-converting enzyme inhibition on diabetic nephropathy. *N Engl J Med* 329: 1456–1462

52 The EUCLIDStudy Group (1997) Randomised placebo-controlled trial of lisinopril in normotensive patients with insulin-dependent diabetes and normoalbuminuria or microalbuminuria. *Lancet* 349: 1787–1792

53 Ravid M, Lang R, Rachmani R, Lishner M (1996) Long-term renoprotective effect of angiotensin-converting enzyme inhibition in non-insulin-dependent diabetes mellitus. *Arch Intern Med* 156: 286–289

54 Chaturvedi N, Sjolie AK, Stephenson JM, Abrahamian H, Keipes M, Castellarin A, Rogulja-Pepeonik Z, Fuller JH, the EUCLIDStudy Group (1998) Effect of lisinopril on progression of retinopathy in normotensive people with type 1 diabetes. *Lancet* 351: 28–31

55 Penno G, Chaturvedi N, Talmud PJ, Cotroneo P, Manto A, Nannipieri M, Luong LA, Fuller JH, the EUCLIDStudy Group (1998) Effect of angiotensin-converting enzyme (ACE) gene polymorphism on progression of renal disease and the influence of ACE inhibition in IDDM patients. *Diabetes* 47: 1507–1511

56 Harjai KJ (1999) Potential new cardiovascular risk factors: Left ventricular hypertrophy, homocysteine, lipoprotein (a), triglycerides, oxidative stress, and fibrinogen. *Ann Intern Med* 131: 376–386

57 McLenachan JM, Henderson E, Morris KI, Dargie HJ (1987) Ventricular arrhythmias in patients with hypertensive left ventricular hypertrophy. *N Engl J Med* 317: 787–792

58 Koren MJ, Savage DD, Casale PN, Laragh JH, Devereux RB (1990) Changes in left ventricular mass predict risk in essential hypertension. *Circulation* 82 (suppl): III-29

59 Dahlöf B (1990) Regression of cardiovascular structural changes – a preventive strategy. *Clin Exp Hypertension* 12 (5): 877–896

60 Dahlöf B, Pennert K, Hansson L (1992) Reversal of left ventricular hypertrophy in hypertensive patients. *Amer J Hypertens* 5: 95–110

61 Schmieder RE, Martus P, Klingbeil A (1996) Reversal of left ventricular hypertrophy in essential hypertension. *JAMA* 275: 1507–1513

62 Jennings G, Wong J (1998) Regression of left ventricular hypertrophy in hypertension: Changing patterns with successive meta-analysis. *J Hypertension* 16 (suppl 6): S29–S34

63 Liebson PR, Grandits GA, Dianzumba S, Princas RJ, Grimm RHJr Neaton JD, Stamler J for the Treatment of Hypertension Study Research Group (1995) Comparison of five antihypertensive monotherapies and placebo for change in left ventricular mass in patients receiving nutritional-hygienic therapy in the treatment of mild hypertension study (TOMHS). *Circulation* 91: 698–706

64 Lièvre M, Guéret P, Gayet C, Roudaut R, Haugh MC, Delair S, Boissel JP on behalf of the HYCARStudy Group (1995) Ramipril-induced regression of left ventricular hypertrophy in treated hypertensive individuals. *Hypertension* 25: 92–97

65 Agabiti-Rosei E, Ambrosioni E, Dal Palu C, Muiesan ML, Zanchetti A (1995) ACE inhibitor ramipril is more effective than the beta-blocker atenolol in reducing left ventricular mass in hypertension. Results of the RACE (ramipril cardioprotective evaluation) study on behalf of the RACE study group. *J Hypertension* 13 (11): 1325–1334

66 Gottdiener JS, Reda DJ, Massie BM, Materson BJ, Williams DW, Anderson RJ for the

VACooperative Study Group on Antihypertensive Agents (1997) Effect of single-drug therapy on reduction of left ventricular mass in mild to moderate hypertension. *Circulation* 95: 2007–2014

67 Devereux RB, Dahlöf B, Levy D, Pfeffer MA (1996) Comparison of enalapril *versus* nifedipine to decrease left ventricular hypertrophy in systemic hypertension (The PRESERVE Trial). *Amer J Cardiol* 78: 61–65

68 Burgess E (1999) Comparative treatment to slow deterioration of renal function: Evidence-based recommendations. *Kidney Int* 55 (suppl 70): S17–S25

69 Giatras I, Lau J, Levey AS for the Angiotensin-Converting-Enzyme Inhibition, Progressive Renal Disease Study Group (1997) Effect of angiotensin-converting enzyme inhibitors on the progression of nondiabetic renal disease: A meta-analysis of randomized trials. *Ann Intern Med* 127: 337–345

70 Zucchelli P, Zuccalà A, Borghi M, Fusaroli M, Sasdelli M, Stallone C, Sanna G, Gaggi R (1992) Long-term comparison between captopril and nifedipine in the progression of renal insufficiency. *Kidney Int* 42: 452–458

71 Hannedouche T, Landais P, Goldfarb B, El Esper N, Fournier A, Godin M, Durand D, Chanard J, Mignon F, Suc JM, Grünfeld JP (1994) Randomised controlled trial of enalapril and β blockers in non-diabetic chronic renal failure. *BMJ* 309: 833–836

72 Maschio G, Alberti D, Janin G, Locatelli F, Mann JFE, Motolese M, Ponticelli C, Ritz E, Zucchelli P, the Angiotensin-Converting-Enzyme Inhibition in Progressive Renal Insufficiency Study Group (1996) Effect of the angiotensin-converting enzyme inhibitor benazepril on the progression of chronic renal insufficiency. *N Engl J Med* 334: 939–945

73 The GISENGroup (1997) Randomised placebo-controlled trial of effect of ramipril on decline in glomerular filtration rate and risk of terminal renal failure in proteinuric, non-diabetic nephropathy. *Lancet* 349: 1857–1863

74 Ruggenenti P, Perna A, Gherardi G, Gaspari F, Benini R, Remuzzi G on behalf of the GISENGroup (1998) Renal function and requirement for dialysis in chronic nephropathy patients on long-term ramipril: REIN follow-up trial. *Lancet* 352: 1252–1256

75 Pfeffer MA, Domanski M, Rosenberg Y, Verter J, Geller N, Albert P, Hsia J, Braunwald E (1998) Prevention of events with angiotensin-converting enzyme inhibition (The PEACE Study Design). *Amer J Cardiol* 82: 25H–30H

76 Teo KK, Burton JR, Buller C, Plante S, Yokoyama S, Montague TJ (1997) Rationale and design features of a clinical trial examining the effects of cholesterol lowering and angiotensin-converting enzyme inhibition on coronary atherosclerosis: Simvastatin/Enalapril Coronary Atherosclerosis Trial (SCAT). *Can J Cardiol* 13 (6): 591–599

77 Fox KM, Henderson JR, Bertrand ME, Ferrari R, Remme WJ, Simoons ML (1998) The European trial on reduction of cardiac events with perindopril in stable coronary artery disease (EUROPA). *Eur Heart J* 19 (suppl J): J52–J55

78 Passa P, Chatellier G (1996) The DIAB-HYCAR Study. *Diabetologia* 39 (12): 1662–1667

79 PROGRESSManagement Committee – Perindopril Protection Against Recurrent Stroke Study (1996) Blood pressure lowering for the secondary prevention of stroke: Rationale and design for PROGRESS. *J Hypertension* 14 (2): S41–S45

80 Yusuf S, Sleight P, Dagenais G, Montague T, Bosch J, Pogue J, Taylor W, Sardo L (2000) Effects of angiotensin-converting enzyme inhibitor, Ramipril, on cardiovascular events in high risk patients. *N Engl J Med* 342 (3): 145–153

81 Golan L, Birkmeyer JD, Welch HG (1999) The cost-effectiveness of treating all patients with type 2 diabetes with angiotensin-converting enzyme inhibitors. *Ann Intern Med* 131: 660–667

The role of ACE inhibition in heart failure

Irene Gavras and Haralambos Gavras

Hypertension and Atherosclerosis Section, Department of Medicine, Boston University School of Medicine, Boston, MA 02118, USA

Introduction

In the early 1970s, ACE inhibition was viewed as an effective means to block the renin-angiotensin component contributing to the maintenance of vasoconstriction [1]. Earlier work had already demonstrated the activation of the renin angiotensin system (RAS) in decompensated congestive heart failure (CHF) [2, 3] and its implications in terms of increased hemodynamic burden to the failing heart. A pilot study using an angiotensin II (Ang II) receptor blocker, saralasin, in a short clinical experiment, demonstrated that Ang II blockade could successfully reverse the hemodynamic aberrations of decompensated CHF, while improving myocardial economy [4]. The decrease in myocardial oxygen consumption resulting from the fall in systemic vascular resistance was, paradoxically, accompanied by an increase in coronary blood flow, a fact that goes against the principles governing the regulation of coronary blood flow. This surprising observation was subsequently explained by the finding that the vasculature of vital organs (heart, kidney and brain) is particularly sensitive to the vasoconstrictive action of Ang II. Consequently, unlike other pharmacological vasodilators, RAS inhibition results in a preferential vasodilation of the coronary, renal and cerebral vasculature, thus maintaining or improving perfusion of vital organs, even in the face of falling systemic blood pressure [5, 6].

From this background knowledge, ACE inhibition evolved as the next logical step in the treatment of CHF. The first clinical trial [7], using the intravenous ACE inhibitor teprotide, confirmed and amplified the results of saralasin, and was followed by similar trials on normotensives and hypertensives with heart failure, with or without coronary artery disease [8–11]. Other studies extended the findings to the newly introduced first oral ACE inhibitor, captopril [9, 12, 13]. Subsequent larger, controlled, longitudinal trials, using various "second generation" ACE inhibitors (see below), further clarified additional properties of this treatment and established the fact that these properties are shared by all these agents and therefore are a class effect of ACE inhibition.

A remarkable aspect of this story is that demonstration of beneficial clinical outcomes preceded, and, indeed, spurred the basic research that subsequently uncovered the multifaceted mechanisms underlying these outcomes.

The following is a brief overview of these mechanisms and a synopsis of the controlled clinical trials that established ACE inhibition as a mandatory treatment for chronic CHF throughout all its stages, i.e., from subclinical diastolic dysfunction to advanced decompensated pump failure.

Pharmacodynamics of ACE inhibition in heart failure

Heart failure is characterized by activation of several neurohumoral factors, including the RAS, the sympathetic nervous system, vasopressin, atrial natriuretic factor(s), endothelin, etc. [14]. It is now accepted that the degree of activation of these factors has both a prognostic value and a pathogenic role contributing to the inexorable progression of CHF [15]. Accumulating evidence indicates that (unlike the standard diuretic and inotropic therapy), inhibition of these factors not only corrects hemodynamic aberrations and relieves symptoms, but can also modify the underlying disease process, thus retarding its progression and improving its outcomes. The first intervention proven to have such effects was ACE inhibition.

Because the ACE acts on both the RAS and the kinin systems, the cardiac (and other) effects of its inhibition are attributable partly to withdrawal of Ang II and partly to potentiation of bradykinin [16]. Both are vasoactive hormones with systemic effects on the general circulation and the regional vasculature of selected organs; and both act also locally as "tissue hormones," either directly on cell structures or by eliciting release of other humoral mediators. Table 1 summarizes some of the systemic and tissue-specific effects of Ang II, which are exerted via stimulation of its AT_1 receptors.

Ang II promotes left ventricular hypertrophy and remodeling both via increase of peripheral resistance and ensuing pressure overload and via direct

Table 1. Actions of angiotensin II via AT_1 receptor stimulation

---

Systemic (endocrine) effects of circulating Ang II
- Vasoconstrictive (preferentially coronary, renal, cerebral)
- Steroidogenic (aldosterone)
- Dipsogenic (CNS effect)
- Renin-suppressing (negative feedback)

Tissue-specific effects of Ang II as local hormone
- Trophic/mitogenic (cardiac and vascular myocytes, fibroblasts)
- Inotropic/contractile (cardiomyocytes)
- Chronotropic/arrhythmogenic (cardiomyocytes)
- Thrombogenic (plasminogen activator inhibitor)
- Oxidative (generation of reactive oxygen species)
- Ion transport channels (myocytes, renal cells)
- Neuroexcitation (sympathetic nerve terminals)
- Endothelin stimulation (endothelial cells)
- Vasopressin stimulation (CNS)

AT_1-mediated actions on cardiomyocytes and adjacent cells, such as fibroblasts. The latter actions include release of numerous growth factors, which act in an autocrine/paracrine fashion to activate enzymes and genes that induce protein and DNA synthesis, such as the transforming growth factor beta$_1$, basic fibroblast growth factor, insulin-like growth factor, etc. [17, 18]. Ang II *per se* can also act as a peptide growth factor in an autocrine/paracrine manner, stimulating the expression of genes that regulate cell growth and proliferation [17, 18]. Finally, Ang II stimulates release of other local hormones, e.g., norepinephrine and endothelin, which possess trophic and mitogenic (as well as inotropic and chronotropic) properties of their own.

Activation of AT_1 receptors in cardiomyocytes triggers also a series of intracellular responses, including calcium mobilization, alteration of ion channels and expression of cytoplasmic proteins. These changes increase the contractility [19] and the conduction velocity of electrical signals [20], thus explaining the positive inotropic and chronotropic actions of Ang II. An inhibitory action of Ang II on cardiac vagal afferents in the central nervous system has also been reported [21].

Withdrawal of these effects when formation of Ang II is suppressed by ACE inhibition in patients with CHF leads to an immediate fall in systemic vascular resistance, pulmonary vascular resistance, pulmonary capillary wedge pressure and heart rate, with increases in stroke volume and cardiac output [7, 9, 10]. The fall in both preload and afterload improves myocardial work indices and energy consumption and is followed by the well-known negative inotropic [22] and chronotropic [23] consequences and the reversal of cardiac hypertrophy associated [29] with sustained ACE inhibition. These effects not only favor cardiac economy, but also result in an important antiarrhythmic influence [25]. Indeed, myocardial irritability and disequilibrium between sympathetic and parasympathetic influences is one of the characteristics of decompensated CHF and is incriminated in part for the high rate of malignant ventricular arrhythmias and sudden deaths that are characteristic of CHF [26]. ACE inhibitors increase the refractory period of cardiomyocytes [23], attenuate the sympathetic stimulation [27] and tend to restore parasympathetic restraint.

Potentiation of bradykinin is another important consequence of ACE inhibition. Bradykinin has a very short half-life and hence a lesser impact on systemic vascular resistance. Its physiologically significant effects are exerted via activation of its B_2-receptor [28]. Use of bradykinin antibodies [29] or selective B_2–receptor antagonists, along with ACE inhibition in experimental studies, suggests that in severe renin-dependent hypertension, about 30% of the blood pressure lowering effect of the ACE inhibitors may be attributable to bradykinin [30–31]. More important may be the regional blood flow alterations within sensitive organs, that may contribute to its cardioprotective and nephroprotective properties. For example, bradykinin causes a redistribution of myocardial blood flow with enhanced perfusion of subendocardial regions at the expense of outer layers of the cardiac muscle [32]; likewise, it causes

Table 2 – Bradykinin-mediated effects of ACE inhibition

- Protection of myocardium from injury of ischemia/reperfusion
- Enhanced perfusion of vulnerable organ regions
- Improved glucose transport and metabolism
- Release of autacoids (nitric oxide, prostacyclin)
- Antimitotic/antiproliferative effects
- Antioxidant activity
- Antithrombotic activity
- Antiarrhythmic action

enhanced perfusion of the papillary areas of the kidney, at the expense of other regions of the renal cortex [33]. These changes are of more than theoretical interest, because the subendocardial region is particularly prone to ischemia in hypertension and the papillary region is particularly prone to ischemic damage from cyclooxygenase inhibitors (e.g., non-steroidal anti-inflammatory drugs).

Table 2 lists some of the currently known B_2-mediated effects of bradykinin that are relevant to myocardial perfusion and metabolism. In addition to its direct B_2-receptor-mediated effects, bradykinin exerts also indirect effects mediated via stimulation of other paracrine factors, mostly from the vascular endothelium, such as nitric oxide and prostaglandins [34, 35]. Indeed, the vasodilatory, antimitotic, antiplatelet and antioxidant properties of bradykinin are, to a large extent, attributable to these autacoids [36–38]. On the contrary, the enhanced insulin-dependent glucose transport and uptake by myocytes and adipocytes is a direct B_2-receptor-mediated effect of bradykinin [39]. This effect explains the clinically observed improvement in insulin sensitivity when essential hypertension, which is characterized by varying degrees of insulin resistance, is treated by ACE inhibitors [40].

The metabolic properties of bradykinin, whether direct or mediated via release of prostacyclin and nitric oxide, contribute to a large extent to the tissue-protective actions of ACE inhibition. These actions are particularly important under conditions of acute or chronic myocardial ischemia and during reperfusion of the infarcted area of the myocardium post-thrombolysis, where ACE inhibitors have been shown to prevent or minimize myocardial dysfunction and injury [41, 42]. Infusion of a bradykinin antagonist could virtually abolish the benefits of concurrent ACE inhibition in terms of both cellular integrity and electrophysiological stability [43].

The putative contribution of bradykinin to the antiarrhythmic effect of ACE inhibition is complex, as bradykinin is known to possess a direct antiarrhythmic property [44] but is also known to cause sympathoexcitation [45, 46] and hence may also exert an indirect proarrhythmic effect. However, the fact that a B_2-receptor antagonist can abolish to a large extent the antiarrhythmic effect of ACE inhibition [43, 47] suggests that the sum of bradykinin's effects favor an antiarrhythmic influence. Ang II blockade on the other hand is unequivocally antiarrhythmic [48] and the fact that chronic therapy with ACE inhibition diminishes the rate of arrhythmias has been well established by numerous experimental and clinical studies [25].

Evidence from longitudinal multicenter trials of ACE inhibition in the treatment of heart failure

Once the acute hemodynamic and functional improvement of CHF by ACE inhibition was established by small clinical studies of short duration [7–10, 49], it was followed by a few more protracted studies that confirmed the sustained effectiveness of this treatment [12, 13, 50]. Subsequently, large multicenter long-term trials were organized to demonstrate the impact of these effects on patient outcomes, i.e., frequency of hospitalizations, rates of recurrence of acute episodes and overall rates of mortality. In parallel, an experimental study in rats demonstrated that chronic ACE inhibition after an acute myocardial infarct (MI) could prevent or retard the progression of myocardial remodeling and left ventricular enlargement and attenuate the progression to CHF [51]. Two clinical trials in post-MI patients corroborated these findings and suggested that initiation of treatment was indicated before appearance of clinical symptoms of CHF [52, 53].

The first large randomized, controlled multicenter trials of ACE inhibition in heart failure were the Captopril Multicenter Research Group and the CONSENSUS trial with enalapril, which found that ACE inhibitors decreased the mortality of patients with severe CHF by up to 40% [54, 55]. The SAVE trial, utilizing captopril in asymptomatic post-MI patients, with left ventricular dysfunction found an overall decrease in mortality by 19% [56]. The SOLVD trial, utilizing enalapril in patients with various degrees of severity of CHF, showed a lesser, but still highly significant reduction in overall mortality by 16% and a more impressive reduction in cardiovascular events by 40% in comparison to placebo [57, 58]. The V-HeFT II trial, comparing enalapril to other vasodilators (with no placebo arm), showed also a significantly reduced mortality from CHF with enalapril by 33.6%, 28.2%, 14% and 10.3% after 1, 2, 3, and 4 years, respectively [59].

Subsequent similar trials were conducted with various other ACE inhibitors, usually in post-MI patients with or without clinical symptomatology of CHF, such as the AIRE trial with ramipril which at six months showed a 27% reduction in total mortality *versus* placebo [60] and its five-year extension, the AIREX, which showed a continuing advantage of treatment [61]; the SMILE trial with zofenopril which showed a 29% decrease in mortality at one year [62]; the GISSI-3 trial with lisinopril which showed a 12% reduction of mortality by six weeks, with continuing divergence of survival curves [63]; the TRACE trial with trandolapril which showed a 22% decrease in total mortality at four years [64]; and other ongoing trials. All have consistently reported significant reduction in overall morbidity and mortality, varying, as expected, with the degree of severity of the disease, i.e., in severely decompensated patients mortality decreased by up to 40%, whereas in modestly affected subjects, the reductions were in the range of 10–15%. A retrospective analysis of 32 trials with seven different ACE inhibitors comprising 7105 patients treated for at least eight weeks, reported a decrease in overall mortality by 23% and in the combined endpoint of mortality or hospitalization by 35% [65]. Another consistent finding has been the decrease in rates of reinfarction or new-onset MI, which dropped by 20–25% [56, 58, 60]. This prompted the initiation of trials where patients with angiographically proven coronary artery disease, but not yet evidence of left ventricular dysfunction, are treated with ACE inhibition in the hope of achieving secondary prevention of ischemic heart disease, such as the QUIET trial with quinapril [66]. A recent retrospective analysis of about 100,000 patients enrolled in various post-MI trials, reported that early initiation and short-term (4–6 weeks) use of ACE inhibitors resulted in a 7% reduction in mortality [67]. Furthermore, the survival benefits appear to be sustained over many years, as the divergence in the mortality curves continues to widen with long-term follow up.

Conclusions

The introduction of ACE inhibitors for treatment of heart failure is one of the most important advances in cardiovascular pharmacology in the last two decades. Cardiomyopathies of all causes appear to benefit from this treatment, but ischemic cardiomyopathy derives the greatest advantage from the hemodynamic and metabolic consequences of both the suppression of Ang II and the potentiation of bradykinin. These effects are due to a multitude of hemodynamic, metabolic, biochemical and cellular mechanisms, some of which are still being explored by ongoing research. Although new aspects of the pathophysiology and molecular biology of ACE inhibition continue to emerge, its therapeutic consequences in terms of improved patient survival and reduction of cardiovascular events are now firmly established on the basis of outcomes from large, randomized, controlled clinical trials. Thus, this treatment is now considered mandatory for heart failure at all stages, its only limitation being intolerance due to side-effects (usually cough, rarely functional renal insufficiency or angioedema and allergic reactions).

References

1 Gavras H, Brunner HR, Laragh JH, Sealey JE, Gavras I, Vukovich RA (1974) An angiotensin converting enzyme inhibitor to identify and treat vasoconstrictor and volume factors in hypertensive patients. *N Engl J Med* 291: 817–821
2 Genest J, Granger A, de Champlain J, Boucher R (1968) Endocrine factors in congestive heart failure. *Amer J Cardiol* 22: 35–42
3 Brown JJ, Davies DL, Johnson VW, Lever AF, Robertson JS (1970) Renin relationship in congestive heart failure, treated and untreated. *Amer Heart J* 80: 329–342

4 Gavras H, Flessas A, Ryan TJ, Brunner HR, Faxon DP, Gavras I (1977) Angiotensin II inhibition: treatment of congestive cardiac failure in a high-renin hypertension. *J Amer Med Assn* 238: 880–882, 1977

5 Liang C, Gavras H, Hood WBJr, (1978) Renin-angiotensin system inhibition in conscious sodium-depleted dogs: Effects on systemic and coronary hemodynamics. *J Clin Invest* 61: 874–883

6 Gavras H, Liang C, Brunner HR (1978) Redistribution of regional blood flow after inhibition of the angiotensin converting enzyme. *Circ Res* 43 (suppl I): I-59–I-63

7 Gavras H, Faxon DP, Berkoben J, Brunner HR, Ryan TJ (1978) Angiotensin converting enzyme inhibition in patients with congestive heart failure. *Circulation* 58: 770–775

8 Turini GA, Brunner HR, Ferguson RK, Rivier JL, Gavras H (1978) Congestive heart failure in normotensive man: hemodynamics, renin and angiotensin II blockade. *Brit Heart J* 40: 1134–1142

9 Turini GA, Brunner HR, Gribic M, Waeber B, Gavras H (1979) Improvement of chronic congestive heart failure by oral captopril. *Lancet* I: 1213–1215

10 Faxon DP, Creager MA, Halperin JL, Gavras H, Coffman JD, Ryan TJ (1980) Central and peripheral hemodynamic effects of angiotensin Inhibition in patients with refractory congestive heart failure. *Circulation* 61: 925–931

11 Faxon DP, Creager MA, Halperin JL, Sussman HA, Gavras H, Ryan TJ (1982) The effect of angiotensin converting enzyme inhibition on coronary blood flow and hemodynamics in patients without coronary artery disease. *Int J Cardiol* 2: 251–262

12 Davis R, Ribner HS, Keung E, Sonnenblick EH, LeJemtel TH (1979) Treatment of chronic heart failure with captopril, an oral inhibitor of angiotensin-converting enzyme. *N Engl J Med* 301: 117–121

13 Levine TB, Franciosa JA, Cohn JA (1980) Acute and long-term response to an oral converting enzyme inhibitor, captopril, in congestive heart failure. *Circulation* 62: 35–41

14 Francis GS, Goldsmith SR, Levine B, Olivan MT, Cohn JN (1984) The neurohumoral axis in congestive heart failure. *Ann Intern Med* 101: 370–377

15 Vantrimpont P, Rouleau JL, Ciampi A, Harel F, de Champlain J, the SAVE investigators (1998) Two-year time course and significance of neurohumoral activation in the SAVE study. *Eur Heart J* 19: 1552–1563

16 Gavras H (1994) Angiotensin-converting enzyme inhibition and the heart. *Hypertension* 23: 813–818

17 Lindpaintner K, Ganten D (1991) The cardiac renin-angiotensin system. *Circ Res* 68: 905–921

18 Dostal DEBaker KM (1995) Biochemistry, molecular biology, and potential roles of the cardiac renin–angiotensin system. *In*: NS Dhalla, N Takeda N, Nagano M (eds): *The Failing Heart*. Lippincott-Raven Publishers, Philadelphia, PA, 275–294

19 Kobayashi M, Furukawa Y, Chiba S (1978) Positive chronotropic and inotropic effects of angiotensin II in the dog heart. *Eur J Pharmacol* 50: 17–25

20 De Mello WC (1996) Renin-angiotensin system and cell communication in the failing heart. *Hypertension* 27: 1267–1272

21 Lee WB, Ismay MJLumbers ER (1980) Mechanisms by which angiotensin affects the heart rate of the conscious sheep. *Circ Res* 47: 286–292

22 Foult JM, Travalaro O, Autony I, Nittenberg A (1988) Direct myocardial and coronary effects of enalaprilat in patient with dilated cardiomyopathy; assessment by a bilateral intracoronary infusion technique. *Circulation* 77: 337–344

23 De Mello WC, Crespo MJ, Altieri PI (1992) Enalapril increases cardiac refractoriness. *J Cardiovasc Pharmacol* 20: 820–825

24 Owens GK (1985) Differential effects of antihypertensive therapy on vascular smooth muscle cell hypertrophy, hyperploidy and hyperplasia in the spontaneously hypertensive rat. *Circ Res* 56: 525–536

25 Wesseling H, De Graeff PA, Van Gilst WH, Kingma JH, De Langen CD (1989 Cardiac arrhythmias: a new indication for angiotensin-converting enzyme inhibitors? *J Hum Hypertens* 3 (suppl 1): 89–95

26 Ponikowski P, Auker SD, Amadi A, Chua TP, Cerquetain D, Ondusova D, O'Sullivan C, Adamopoulos S, Piepoli MCoats AJS (1996) Heart rhythms, ventricular arrhythmias and death in chronic heart failure. *J Cardiac Fail* 2: 1772–1783

27 Carlsson LAbrahamsson T (1989) Ramiprilat attenuates the local release of noradrenaline in the ischemic myocardium. *Eur J Pharmacol* 166: 157–164

28 Regoli D (1986) Kinins, receptors, antagonists. *Adv Exp Med Biol* 198: 549–558
29 Carretero OA, Miyazaki S, Scicli AG (1981) Role of kinins in the acute antihypertensive effect of the converting enzyme inhibitor captopril. *Hypertension* 3: 18–22
30 Benetos A, Gavras H, Stewart JM, Vavrek RJ, Hatinoglou S, Gavras I (1986) Vasodepressor role of endogenous bradykinin assessed by a bradykinin antagonist. *Hypertension* 8: 971–974
31 Bao G, Gohlke P, Qadri F, Unger T (1992) Chronic kinin receptor blockade attentuates the antihypertensive effect of ramipril. *Hypertension* 20: 74–79
32 Ruocco NAJr Bergelson BA, Yu T-K, Gavras I, Gavras H (1995) Augmentation of coronary blood flow by ACE: Role of angiotensin and bradykinin. Clin Exper Hypertens 17: 1059–1072
33 Fenoy FJ, Scicli AG, Carretero O, Roman RJ (1991) Effect of an angiotensin II and a kinin receptor antagonist on he renal hemodynamic response to captopril. *Hypertension* 17: 1038–1044
34 McGiff JC, Itkoviz HD, Terragno A, Wong PYK (1976) Modulation and mediation of the action of the renal kallikrein-system by prostaglandins. *Fed Proc* 35: 175–180
35 Weimer G, Scholkens BA, Becker RHA, Busse R (1991) Ramiprilat enhances endothelial-autacoid formation by inhibiting breakdown of endothelium-derived bradykinin. *Hypertension* 18: 558–563
36 Wang Y-X, Gavras I, Wierzba T, Lammek B, Gavras H (1992) Inhibition of nitric oxide, bradykinin, and prostaglandins in normal rats. *Hypertension* 19 (suppl II): 255–261
37 Moncada S, Palmer RMJ, Higgs EA (1991) Nitric oxide: physiology, pathophysiology and pharmacology. *Pharmacol Rev* 43: 109–142
38 Islim IF, Beevers DG, Bareford D (1992) The effect of antihypertensive drugs on *in vivo* platelet activity in essential hypertension. *J Hypertension* 10: 379–383
39 Kohlman O Jr, De Assis Rocha Neves F, Ginoza M, Tavares A, Cezaretti ML, Zanella MT, Ribeiro AB, Gavras I, Gavras H (1995) Role of bradykinin in insulin sensitivity and blood pressure regulation during hyperinsulinemia. *Hypertension* 25: 1003–1007
40 Tomiyama H, Kushiro T, Abeta H, Islin T, Takahashi A, Furukawa I Asagami T, Hino T, Saito F, Otsuka Yet al (1994) Kinins contribute to the improvement of insulin sensitivity during treament with angiotensin converting enzyme inhibitor. *Hypertension* 23: 450–455
41 Li K, Chen X (1987) Protective effects of captopril and enalapril on myocardial ischemia and reperfusion damage of rat. *J Mol Cell Cardiol* 19: 909–915
42 Tio RA, De Langen CDJ, De Graeff PA, Van Gilst WH, Bel KJ, Wolters KGTP, Mook PH, van Wijngaarden J, Wesseling H (1990) The effects of oral pretreatment with zofenopril, an angiotensin-converting enzyme inhibitor, on early reperfusion and subsequent electrophysiologic stability in the pig. *Cardiovasc Drug Therapy* 4: 695–704
43 Scholkens BA, Linz W, Konig W (1988) Effects of the angiotensin converting enzyme inhibitor ramipril in isolated ischemic rat heart are abolished by a bradykinin antagonist. *J Hypertension* 6 (suppl 4): 525–528
44 Gavras I (1992) Bradykinin-mediated effects of ACE inhibition. *Kidney Int* 42: 1020–1029
45 Staszewska-Barczak J, Van JR (1967) The release of catecholamines from the adrenal medulla by peptides. *Brit J Pharmacol Chemother* 30: 655–667
46 Rump LC, Berlit T, Schwertfeger E, Beyerdorf F, Schollmeyer P, Bohmann C (1997) Angiotensin converting enzyme inhibition unmasks the sympthofacilitatory effect of bradykinin in human right atrium. *J Hypertension* 15: 1263–1270
47 Van Gilst WH, De Graeff PA, Wesseling H, de Langen CDJ (1986) Reduction of reperfusion arrhythmias in the ischemic isolated rat heart by angiotensin converting enzyme inhibitors: A comparison of captopril, enalapril, and HOE498. *J Cardiovasc Pharmacol* 8: 722–728
48 Lee Y-M, Peng Y-Y, Ding Y-A, Yen M-H (1997) Losartan attenuates myocardial ischemia-induced ventricular arrhythmias and reperfusion injury in spontaneously hypertensive rats. *Amer J Hypertens* 10: 852–858
49 Curtiss C, Cohn JN, Vrobel T, Franciosa JA (1978) Role of the renin-angiotensin system in the systemic vasoconstriction of chronic congestive heart failure. *Circulation* 58: 763–770
50 Dzau VJ, Colucci WS, Williams GH, Curfman G, Meggs L, Hollenberg NK (1980) Sustained effectiveness of converting enzyme inhibition in patients with severe congestive heart failure. *N Engl J Med* 302: 1373–1379
51 Pfeffer MA, Pfeffer JA, Steinberg C, Finn P (1985) Survival and experimental myocardial infarction: beneficial effects of long-term therapy with captopril. *Circulation* 72: 406–412
52 Sharpe N, Murphy J, Smith H, Hannan S (1988) Treatment of patients with symptomless left ventricular dysfunction after myocardial infarction. *Lancet* 1: 255–259

53 Pfeffer MA, Lamas GA, Vaughan DE, Paris AF, Braunwald E (1988) Effect of captopril on progressive ventricular dilation after anterior myocardial infarction. *N Engl J Med* 319: 80–86
54 Captopril Multicenter Research Group (1983) A placebo-controlled trial of captopril in refractory chronic congestive heart failure. *J Amer Coll Cardiol* 2: 755–763
55 The CONSENSUSTrial Study Group (1987) Effects of enalapril on mortality in severe congestive heart failure: results of the Cooperative North Scandinavian Enalpril Survival Study (CONSENSUS). *N Engl J Med* 316: 1429–1435
56 Pfeffer MA, Braunwald E, Moye LA, Basta L, Brown EJ, Cuddy TE, Davis BR, Geltman EM, Goldman S, Flater GC et al (1992) Effect of captopril on mortality and morbidity in patients with left ventricular dysfunction after myocardial infarction. Results of the Survival and Ventricular Enlargement Trial. *N Engl J Med* 327: 669–677
57 The SOLVDInvestigators (1991) Effect of enalapril on survival in patients with reduced left ventricular ejection fractions and congestive heart failure. *N Engl J Med* 325: 293–302
58 The SOLVDInvestigators (1992) Effect of enalapril on mortality and the development of heart failure in asymptomatic patients with reduced left ventricular ejection fractions. *N Engl J Med* 327: 685–691
59 Cohn JN, Johnson G, Ziesche S, Cobb F, Francis G, Tristawi F, Smith R, Dunkman B, Loeb H, Wong M et al (1991) A comparison of enalapril with hydralazine-isosorbide dinitrate in the treatment of chronic heart failure. *N Engl J Med* 325: 303–310
60 The Acute Infarction Ramipril Efficacy (AIRE) Study Investigators (1993) Effect of ramipril on mortality and morbidity of survivors of acute myocardial infarction with clinical evidence of heart failure. *Lancet* 342: 821–828
61 Hall AS, Murray GD, Ball SG on behalf of the AIREXStudy Investigators (1997) Follow-up study of patients randomly allocated ramipril or placebo for heart failure after acute myocardial infarction: AIRE Extension (AIREX) study. *Lancet* 349: 1493–1497
62 Ambrosioni E, Borghi C, Magnani B for the Survival of myocardial Infarction Long-term evaluation (SMILE) Study Investigators (1995) The effect of the angiotensin-converting enzyme inhibitor zofenopril on mortality and morbidity after anterior myocardial infarction. *N Engl J Med* 332: 80–85
63 GISSI-3 (Gruppo Italiano per lo Studio della Sopravvivenza nell'Infarto Miocardico) (1994) Effects of lisinopril and transdermal glyceryl trinitrate singly and together on 6-week mortality and ventricular function after acute myocardial infarction. *Lancet* 343: 1115–1122
64 Kober L, Torp-Pedersen C, Carlsen JE, et al for the Trandolapril Cardiac Evaluation (TRACE) Study Group (1995) A clinical trial of the angiotensin-converting enzyme inhibitor trandolapril in patients with left ventricular dysfunction after myocardial infarction. *N Engl J Med* 333: 1670–1676
65 Garg R, Yusuf S (1995) Overview of randomized trials of angiotensin-converting enzyme inhibitors on mortality and morbidity in patients with heart failure. *J Amer Med Assn* 273: 1450–1456
66 Texter M, Lees RS, Pitts B, Dinsmore RE, Uprichard AC (1993) The Quinapril Ischemic Event Trial (QUIET) design and methods; evaluation of chronic ACE inhibitor therapy after coronary artery intervention. *Cardiovasc Drug Ther* 7: 273–282
67 ACE inhibitor Myocardial Infarction Collaborative Group (1998) Indication for ACE inhibitors in the early treatment of acute myocardial infarction: Systematic overview of individual data from 100,000 patients in randomized trials. *Circulation* 97: 2202–2212

ACE Inhibitors
ed. by P. D'Orléans-Juste and G.E. Plante
© 2001 Birkhäuser Verlag/Switzerland

Angiotensin converting enzyme inhibition in the microcirculation

Gérard E. Plante and Tewfik Nawar

Departments of Medicine (Nephrology), Physiology and Pharmacology, Institute of Pharmacology, University of Sherbrooke, Sherbrooke (Québec), Canada

From macro- to microcirculation

Structural characteristics of blood vessels

Microcirculation networks represent highly specialized segments of the general circulation in terms of structure and function. Definition of these segments is critical to establish the volume of blood contained, the endothelial surface exposed to the neighbouring fluid compartments, including the interstitial and cellular compartments, the lumen diameter and wall thickness of each segment. In fact, these structural characteristics determine a large part of the physiological functions of the vasculature, from hydrostatic pressure development to fluid and nutrient exchanges in peripheral organs.

The high pressure system includes the thoracic and abdominal aorta, followed by the large distribution arteries and the terminal arterioles which are subdivided into three types based on their specific size, from 60.5 to 14.8 µm, and tonus. The high pressure system is responsible for blood delivery to peripheral organs but contains under normal conditions only 11% of the total blood volume, the smallest fraction. The approximate cross-sectional area of this segment is 425 cm^2, the wall thickness decreases from 2 mm to 20 µm and the lumen diameter similarly diminishes from 2.5 cm to 30 µm.

The low pressure system includes capillaries, post-capillary venules, collecting and larger central veins, as well as the entire pulmonary circulation, both arterial and venous. Methods used to measure the volume of blood contained in the microcirculation make it difficult to quantify precisely the contribution of capillary and post-capillary venule segments. It is evident, however, that the largest fraction of the vascular volume is contained in the microcirculation, most likely in the range of 35 to 40%. The total cross-sectional area of capillaries and post-capillary venules averages 8,500 cm^2. The wall thickness is similar, 1 to 2 µm, while the lumen diameter ranges from 5 to 20 µm in these two segments of the microcirculation. Finally, the collecting and larger veins contain between 15 and 20% of the total blood volume, while their cross-sectional area is rather low, 40 and 18 cm^2, respectively. The wall thickness in these two segments increases from 0.5 mm to 1.5 mm, while their lumen diameter rises from 0.5 to 3 cm, respectively [1].

Lymphatic circulation

The lymphatic circulation is responsible for the drainage of the interstitial compartments, in particular the washout of albumin that escapes recovery by the microcirculation and some structural macromolecules such as glycosaminoglycans [2]. The lymph vessels traverse lymph nodes and move fluid and solutes back to the central venous circulation by episodic contraction of their thin wall which resembles capillaries. Lymph propulsion depends on spontaneous contraction of the vessel wall which is influenced by locally-produced vasoactive mediators, including nitric oxide. In contrast to capillaries, the lymph vessel endothelial-like cells have no basement membrane and no intercellular junctions [1].

The structural aspects of the blood and lymph circulation systems briefly presented above have a critical importance on the microcirculation, including rheological features, especially at the level of arterial division. For instance, the right angle pattern of renal interlobar, arcuate and interlobular arteries is responsible for the plasma skimming phenomenon. In addition, the way blood reaches the microcirculation networks from the delivery arteries and resistance arterioles, as well as the way collecting and larger veins remove that blood from post-capillary venules, will have a major impact on the microcirculation beds. Similarly, drainage of interstitial compartments by the lymphatic circulation, and metabolism of structural macromolecules contained in this compartment will also influence the microcirculation dynamics. Pre-capillary resistances, particularly in poorly autoregulated microcirculation networks, due to disease processes or pharmacological interventions, will affect the velocity of laminar blood flow and create turbulence which may in turn affect endothelial structure and function downstream. Such phenomena have been elegantly documented by Kiani et al. at bifurcation of microvessels [3], and by Davies in endothelial cell culture preparations [4].

Ultrastructure of the microcirculation

The structure of capillary and post-capillary venules is also of primary importance to understanding how fluid, small solutes, and macromolecules move across the endothelial barrier, from the vascular to the interstitial compartments and *vice versa*. As in most living organisms and biological systems, the endothelial structure of microcirculation networks in mammalian species is markedly heterogeneous. Basically, the endothelial cells sit on a continuous basement membrane containing glycosaminoglycans, as in epithelia. In most networks, endothelial cells are also tightly bound one to the other by junction complexes and other intercellular structures which allow cell-cell communications, as observed also in epithelia [5]. It is likely that the ultrastructure of junction complexes also differs from one microcirculation network to another, and even within a given organ. On the outer surface of capillaries, pericytes are found in a dispersed fashion, wrapping the vessel wall [1]. These contractile cells have a structural and functional pattern similar to those of the glomerular mesangial cells, and probably contribute to local blood flow regulation, basement membrane and interstitial matrix synthesis [6]. In other networks, the endothelial cells are fenestrated, as in the liver or kidney glomerular network.

These structural characteristics influence the relative permeability characteristics to fluid, small solutes and macromolecules of the different micorcirculation networks. A major impact on some functional characteristics of endothelial cells has been documented by measuring baseline hydraulic conductivity in different networks. This parameter averages 3×10^{-13} $cm^3s^{-1}dyne^{-1}$ in the brain microcirculation, the so-called very tight blood-brain barrier, and $15,000 \times 10^{-13}$ $cm^3s^{-1}dyne^{-1}$ in the kidney glomerular microcirculation, one of the most permeable endothelial networks. The hydraulic conductivity in other areas, where it has been measured, varies from 100 to 860×10^{13} $cm^3s^{-1}dyne^{-1}$, in the skin, skeletal muscle, lung, heart and gastrointestinal mucosa, respectively [1].

Rheological features

The velocity of blood flow varies with respect to the relative resistance of the microcirculation network and begins changing mainly at the level of terminal arterioles where the total cross-sectional area of the blood vessels reaches its highest values. The potential extravasation of fluid, small solutes and macromolecules into the interstitial compartment is highly dependent on the endothelial permeability characteristics in this enormous and heterogeneous cross-sectional area of the vasculature. In addition, and of critical pathophysiological interest, the importance of blood flow reserve, which can be evaluated by measuring blood flow before and after reactive hyperemia in different organs, coincides with high endothelial permeability characteristics. The magnitude of extravasation will peak upon maximum work load imposed on organs such as the heart and the kidney, whereas dissociated features in these parameters will produce opposite effects in other organs, such as the skin and skeletal muscle, as illustrated in Figure 1 [7].

Available methods used to study microcirculation

Methods used to study the physiology, pathophysiology and pharmacology of regional microcirculation networks are relatively limited at this point in time,

BLOOD FLOW RESERVE (%) AND
ENDOTHELIAL BASELINE PERMEABILITY

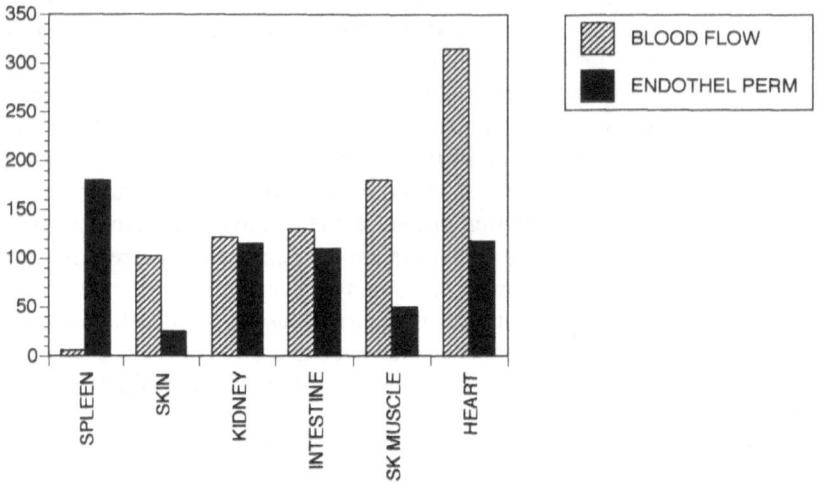

Figure 1. Blood flow reserve (obtained during reactive hyperemia or physiological stimulation) and baseline capillary permeability to Evans blue in peripheral (skin, skeletal muscle), thoracic (heart) and splanchnic (spleen, intestine, kidney) organs. It is of interest to note that the kidney and intestine both have high blood flow reserve and high baseline capillary permeability to Evans blue.

especially for those investigators wishing to use a non-invasive technology. *In vivo* and *in vitro* methods are available to study microcirculation in experimental animals and in human subjects. The *in vitro* approach has the advantage of excluding the contribution of the autonomic nervous system and circulating hormones, which also modulate pre- and post-capillary resistances as well as endothelial permeability.

A number of networks are accessible for *in vivo* studies. The subcutaneous microcirculation is studied in the cheek pouch [8], the mesenteric bed [9], a representative of the splanchnic blood flow. The skeletal muscle [10] is similarly examined in the trapezius and the cremaster preparations. Finally, the cerebral superficial cortex arterioles are available for direct study using serial photomicrography. The size of different arteriolar segments, capillaries and post–capillary venules are directly measured in the rat and hamster models. Micropuncture technology opened the exploration of glomerular blood flow characteristics. The respective roles of hydrostatic and oncotic pressures in the glomerular ultrafiltration process has been established using this methodology [11]. Of course, these methods are limited to a small number of organs, and extrapolation of observations even made in a single organ must be made with caution. As an example, studies performed in the serosal mesenteric microcirculation network are not necessarily representative of what happens in the mucosal side of the gastrointestinal tract [12].

A unique *in vivo* method to look at regional capillary permeability to macro-molecules has been used by us [13], and other laboratories [14], and can be applied to examine this particular microcirculation characteristic in almost all organs. In unanesthetized normal or diseased animals, a bolus of Evans blue is injected in the caudal vein and sacrificed ten min after. Following careful exsanguination, selected organs are rapidly dissected and removed. Evans blue is extracted with formamide and measured by spectrophotometry. The amount of this albumin marker is representative of plasma extravasation into the inter-stitial space, due to combined capillary and post-capillary venule endothelial function. The reproducibility of measurements is remarkable, and the level of contamination due to vascular residual blood is less than 8%, in the highly vas-cularized organs, as shown in Figure 2 [15]. Seasonal variations in capillary permeability to macromolecules have been observed [16]. Therefore, when using this approach to examine regional endothelial permeability it becomes important to perform appropriate time-control experiments. Finally, it is also important to notice that important species differences in regional endothelial permeability have been reported, and include studies performed in the mouse, rat, hamster, rabbit, chicken, and dog. Fluorescence microscopy which turns Evans blue to a red color is another interesting possibility to look at distribu-tion of endothelial permeability changes, such as in large blood vessels (lumi-nal *versus* antiluminal endothelia) or in the kidney (glomerular *versus* per-itubular endothelia) [17].

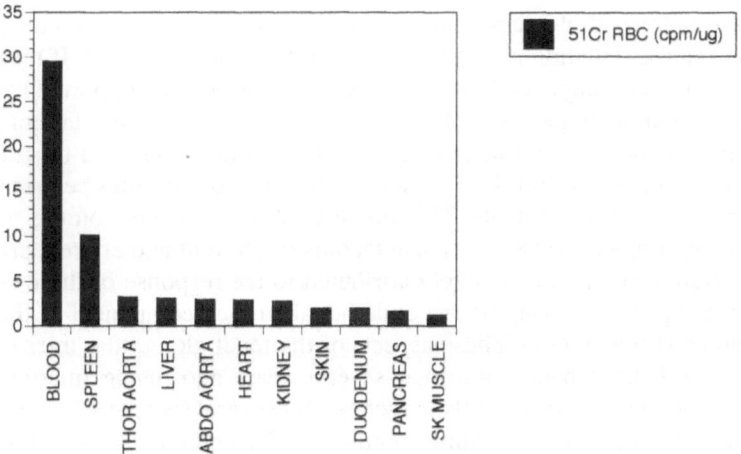

MICROCIRCULATION RESIDUAL BLOOD
FOLLOWING RAT EXSANGUINATION

Figure 2. Residual blood in different microcirculation networks of the vasculature following post sac-rifice exsanguination in normal rats. The maximum absolute and relative blood "contamination" is found in the spleen microcirculation whereas in all other vascular networks examined the residual blood was less than 8%.

For studies in human subjects, different indirect and direct methods are available to look at regional changes in microcirculation, and to evaluate the effects of pharmacological agents. Monitoring of baseline or induced changes in skin temperature, by acute arterial occlusion (post-ischemic hyperemia), has been used successfully. Plethysmography is also being used to look at changes in peripheral blood flow, including both large vessels, skeletal muscle and skin microcirculation networks. More recently, elegant, noninvasive nailfold capillaroscopy allows the direct evaluation of skin microvessels in human subjects. Baseline behavior of microcirculation and the stimulated response (post occlusive hyperemia) of capillaries can be studied [18].

Isolated vascular preparations can be studied *in vitro*, either to look at contractile responses to direct application of vaso-active autacoids, or to examine gene expression of important mediators of microcirculatory responses using molecular biology techniques [19]. Segments of small arteries of different sizes obtained by biopsy material from human volunteers are available for structure-function *in vitro* studies [20]. More recently, complete *vasa vasorum* microcirculation networks carefully dissected from bovine aorta specimens were made available for endothelin-induced contractile response studies [21]. Similarly, we also used the *vasa vasorum* system of the rabbit thoracic aorta to examine the contractile response of pre-capillary arterioles, as well as the endothelial permeability to Evans blue, following stimulation by a variety of vaso-active autacoids [22].

Interpretation of results obtained *in vivo* or *in vitro*, particularly in studies looking at changes in pre- and post-capillary resistances, or looking at the influence of these changes on endothelial permeability in microcirculation networks, may be ambiguous. In fact, in all studies performed at this point in time in this area of microcirculation, the role of pericytes which are distributed between the two strategic resistances mentioned above, mostly on the venous side of microcirculation networks, are completely neglected [6]. If these cells resemble the mesangial cells of the kidney glomerulus, as supported by several ultrastructural studies, it is likely that the pericytes exert similar contractile properties, capable of influencing regional Starling forces, and by extension passive movements of fluid, small solutes and macromolecules between blood and interstitial compartments. The uninterrupted controversy on the selective contractile response to vaso-active autacoids of afferent and efferent arterioles of the kidney glomerulus is likely attributed to the response of these contractile cells capable of changing the endothelial surface component of the ultrafiltration coefficient (Kf). These aspects of the renal glomerular microcirculation network have been confirmed several years ago, using micropuncture technology. The mesangial cells in fact exhibit several receptors to a variety of vaso-active mediators, including angiotensin-II, endothelins, arginine-vasopressin, and prostaglandins [23].

Effect of ACE inhibition on microcirculation

Similarity or heterogeneity of ACE inhibitors

The question of pharmacological homogeneity within the class of angiotensin converting enzyme inhibitors is still pending, and being debated by competitive drug companies. The prototype of this class, captopril, exhibited a SH group that was held responsible for a number of negative side-effects, including taste alteration. Later on, the same chemical SH group was thought to be related to the anti-protease action of the drug because of its zinc chelating effect [24]. Differences in the chemical structure of ACE inhibitors have not yet been reported to produce different actions on angiotensin-II production or bradykinin accumulation, two important pharmacological actions of these drugs. Doses of inhibitors used both in experimental animals and in human subjects could be associated with different responses. It is well-known that sub-pressive doses of angiotensin-II are associated with significant biological effects, as if non-angiotensin-II-dependent pharmacological actions were responsible for these effects, such as increased sulphatation of aortic glycosaminoglycans [25].

Similarly, it is interesting that megadoses of captopril initially used in hypertensive patients were not accompanied by cough, a bradykinin-reputed side-effect, as if bradykinin accumulation failed to develop with these high doses of captopril. However, it is much more evident that the pharmacokinetics of ACE inhibitors is different from one molecule to the other. The concept of tissue penetration, in other words the preferential localization of ACE inhibitors in the microcirculation and/or interstitium of some organs, is of clinical interest because it may provide longer exposition of target tissues to the selective pharmacological actions of the drug [26]. It is of interest that differences in the chemical structure of ACE inhibitors could be responsible for the observed albumin binding of these drugs, and hence their ability to reach their specific target, endothelial cells, vascular smooth muscle cells, or interstitial fibroblasts [27].

ACE inhibition and microcirculation resistances

Several years ago, Vacek and Braveny, using serial photomicrography in the normotensive rat, were able to show regional differences in the mesentery, skin, and skeletal muscle responses to angiotensin-II, in both pre- and post-capillary resistances [28]. Using the cremaster muscle preparation, Meininger et al. were able to establish the hydrostatic pressure profile in different segments of the microcirculation, measured in types 1, 2 and 3 arterioles, as well as in type 3, 2 and 1 venules [29]. If the cremaster muscle is representative of what happens in the whole skeletal muscle mass, values obtained might be of critical importance in studying arterial hypertension since total peripheral resistance develops in this critical organ. As illustrated in Figure 3, there are two major sites of resistance along the microcirculation network: the first site is at the level of type 1 arterioles where the vascular pressure drops from 90 to 40 mmHg, and the second site is between type 3 arterioles and type 3 venules, the capillary component of the microcirculation, where pressure drops again from 40 to 18 mmHg. It is important to notice that capillaries represent a significant component of the so-called peripheral resistance: the 65% pressure drop at this level is almost identical to the 66% drop which occurs between the femoral distribution artery and type 1 arterioles. These findings suggest that what happens in capillaries, and perhaps in the interstitial compartment outside capillaries, might be important in the development of total peripheral resistance in disease states such as essential, salt-dependent, or renovascular arterial hypertension.

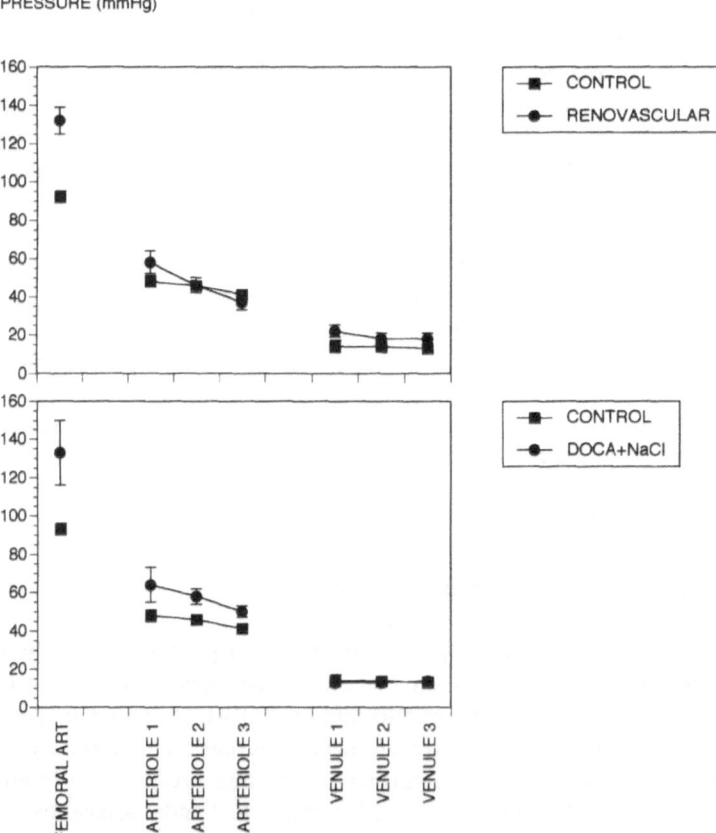

Figure 3. Blood pressure profile in different segments of the vasculature measured in normotensive, salt-sensitive and renovascular hypertensive rats. All values were obtained *in vivo* from measurements taken in the cremaster muscle (modified from [29]).

It is of interest that the pressure drop profile between these two critical resistance sites differs in the spontaneous hypertensive rat (SHR) essential hypertension animal model, in the salt-dependent and in the renovascular type hypertension. In addition, investigators also looked at the pressure profile in other microcirculation networks, such as the intestinal, the kidney, and the cerebral cortex [30]. Heterogeneity in the pattern of pressure drop at both resistance sites were documented, much more though, between terminal arterioles and initial venules, again in the capillary segment of the microcirculation. Heterogeneity was even observed between two networks from the same organ, the mucosal and the visceral microcirculation of the intestine. The significance of this heterogeneous pattern of pressure drop in the vasculature between organs, and between hypertension of different pathophysiology, has not been thoroughly examined. It is likely that the heterogeneous pattern of endothelial permeability and interstitial composition found in the different organs examined could be responsible for the observed findings.

The response of arterioles and venules to vaso-active mediators, including neuromediators, such as norepinephrine and acetylcholine, realeased at autonomic nerve terminals, is enhanced in most types of experimental hypertension and the phenomenon is enhanced with time, at least for angiotensin-II and norepinephrine [31]. In elegant studies performed on the cremaster muscle by Vicaut and Hou, the respective contribution of the systemic and the local angiotensin converting enzyme was examined. At the microvascular level, these authors observed that circulating renin and angiotensinogen levels were more effective in inducing arteriolar constriction than the local system. Angiotensin converting enzyme inhibitors therefore represent potent pharmacological tolls to modulate skeletal muscle microcirculation. Interestingly, these authors also demonstrated that the contractile response to angiotensin-I was of increasing magnitude from second to fourth-order types of arterioles [32]. Using another model, the cheek pouch, the response to angiotensin-II and arginine vasopressin was found to be different at the arteriolar and venous ends of the skin microcirculation. Arginine vasopressin was a more potent vasoconstrictor on the arteriolar side than angiotensin-II, but the latter agonist exhibited a more potent vasoconstriction on the venous side. Using the same model, the authors also observed that the response to both vasoconstrictors was markedly enhanced in the renovascular hypertensive animal [33].

ACE inhibition and capillary rarefaction

A potential consequence of precapillary vasoconstriction appears to be a strange phenomenon called arteriolar or capillary rarefaction, which is now being investigated in relation to the development of arterial hypertension. Is this phenomenon a physiological feature or is it involved only in pathophysiological conditions? Does it precede hypertension or could it be a non-specific consequence of the disease?

Capillary rarefaction has been described as a reduction in capillary density, or in the number of arterioles in a given tissue area. Since blood flow entering this tissue area is delivered in a reduced vascular compartment, pressure increases [34]. Some authors believe that the abnormality is already present in young SHR, before systemic hypertension develops, and consider the phenomenon as defective vasculogenesis [35]. Since capillary rarefaction is also present in non-essential types of hypertension, the abnormality is probably functional in nature. Adrenaline released by sympathetic fibers increases reactivity in terminal arterioles of renovascular hypertensive rats. Since angiotensin-II affects sympathetic activity, it is likely that converting enzyme is involved in the process of capillary rarefaction [36]. The early functional nature of the phenomenon appears to be followed by structural rarefaction. This aspect has been studied in the cremaster muscle preparation in renovascular hypertensive rats at different time periods following induction of hypertension. As shown in Figure 4, the number of terminal arterioles is reduced in all groups at rest, when compared to normotensive rats. In response to adenosine, the number of arterioles that re-opens is normal in the two younger groups, but the older group of hypertensive rats fails to respond [37].

This original way of looking at peripheral resistance being situated so far downstream in the vasculature is not unanimously accepted by scientists

NUMBER OF TERMINAL ARTERIOLES AS
HYPERTENSION DEVELOPS

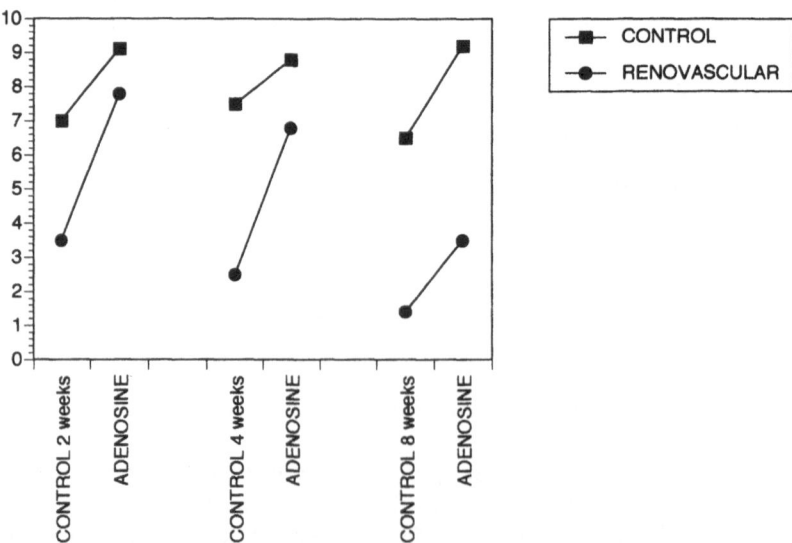

Figure 4. Changes in the number of terminal cremaster arterioles following adenosine in renovascular hypertensive rats. Control and experimental measurements were obtained in animals of different ages (modified from [37]).

involved in the pathophysiology of arterial hypertension. The effect of high-salt intake on microvascular rarefaction in the reduced renal mass rat has been elegantly examined. In this model, microvascular changes developed before elevation of blood pressure and in a context of renin-angiotensin system suppression. Paradoxically, infusion of systemic subpressor doses of angiotensin-II, was associated with normalization of the microvessel density, as illustrated in Figure 5 [38]. The possibility of an extravascular event being responsible for the capillary rarefaction phenomenon has not yet been explored, but certainly deserves scientific interest for two reasons.

First, the pressure gradient, the net hydrostatic and oncotic pressures between intracapillary and interstitial fluid compartment, although difficult to measure, is relatively small under normal conditions and differs from one organ to the other. This gradient normally favors slight net fluid movement towards the interstitial space, in which lymphatic vessels bring a neutral net fluid balance. Under conditions where this neutral balance is disturbed, accumulation of fluid and solutes, including macromolecules such as albumin, is likely to alter interstitial geometry, composition and pressure, which could easily lead to capillary collapse. We have already reported a selective bradykinin-

EFFECT OF LOW-DOSE ANGIOTENSIN-II
ON THE MICROCIRCULATION OF SALT-
SENSITIVE HYPERTENSIVE RATS

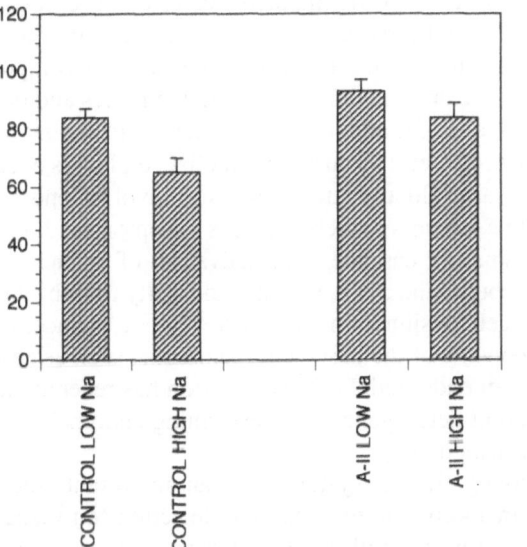

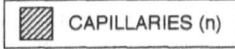 CAPILLARIES (n)

Figure 5. Effect of subpressive angiotensin II infusion on microvessel density in salt-sensitive hypertensive rats. Under normal conditions, where baseline angiotensin II blood levels are low, the number of vessel intersections is reduced both in control and hypertensive rats. Angiotensin II infusion restores the microvessel rarefaction (modified from [38]).

dependent, endothelial dysfunction, characterized by renal albumin extravasation and interstitial swelling, in the four-week SHR rat, before hypertension developed [39]. This finding supports the hypothesis that extravascular phenomena, perhaps initiated by endothelial dysfunction, might be responsible for capillary rarefaction.

Second, the role of interstitial glycosaminoglycans, anionic macromolecules with very hydrophilic and cation-binding capacities [40], has not been largely explored in relation to the development of hypertension. Although present in small quantities, these substances affect the interstitial distribution of albumin, thereby influencing the hydraulic properties of this strategic fluid compartment. In addition, glycosaminoglycans play a role in the developement of interstitial negative pressure. In a recent report, angiotensin-II was shown to modulate the metabolism of these macromolecules: subpressor doses of this peptide augment the sulphatation of glycosaminoglycans [25]. These findings also indicate that interstitial events could be involved in the balance of physical forces maintaining the size and number of small vessels in microcirculation networks.

ACE inhibition and endothelial permeability

Endothelial permeability plays a critical role in microcirculation networks because it determines the size and composition of individual organ interstitial compartments, which are responsible for the maintenance of cell life in these organs. In fact, the movement of vital substrates towards, and removal of waste products from the cell mass, occurs in the interstitium, the size and composition of which is determined by the endothelial function of capillaries and post-capillary venules [41]. The passage of macromolecules, including all albumin-bound substances (hormones, drugs, etc) through endothelial cell layers occurs either by the transcellular or paracellular routes. The latter involves endothelial cell dysjunction, an active process which includes receptor binding of autacoids, an intracellular signaling cascade, and activation of intracellular contractile proteins, such as tubulin and actin, which lead finally to tight-junction-complex alteration and cell dysjunction [42]. The role of extracellular interstitial proteins and components of the basement membrane, such as collagen and glycosaminoglycans, in endothelial cell dysjunction has recently also been identified. Microcirculation heterogeneity in performing endothelial cell dysjunction has also been identified [43].

Components of the renin-angiotensin system play an important role in endothelial cell dysjunction, in addition to their contractile actions on vascular smooth muscle cells of pre- and post-capillary resistances, and likely also on post-capillary venule pericytes. As illustrated in Figure 6, two converting enzyme inhibitors, captopril and perindopril, exhibit different effects on Evans blue extravasation in a variety of microcirculation networks [44]. Performed *in vivo*, and in normal unanesthetized rats, the results indicate two interesting fea-

EVANS BLUE EXTRAVASATION
(ug/g Dry Weight)

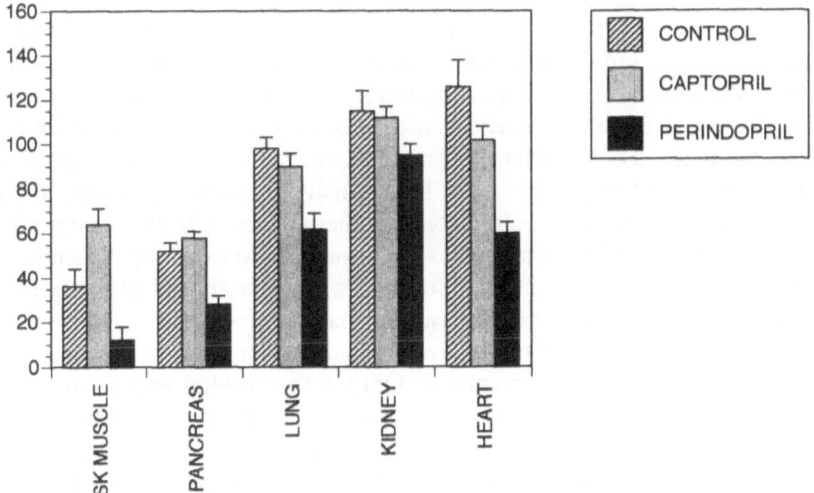

Figure 6. Evans blue extravasation measured in different microcirculation networks in normal unanesthetized rats. The effect of two angiotensin converting enzyme inhibitors on capillary permeability to Evans blue was compared (modified from [44, 45]).

tures. First, as usual, microcirculation networks exhibit heterogeneity in their response, second, the two inhibitors tested show differences, not only in potency, but also in the direction of their pharmacological effects. Captopril increases albumin extravasation in the skin whereas perindopril has the opposite effect. Captopril fails to affect Evans blue leakage in the pancreas, lung parenchyma and kidney, while perindopril reduces endothelial permeability in the same organs. The kidney microcirculation network as a whole, remains unchanged by the two drugs. When captopril is administered with HOE-140, a bradykinin B2-receptor antagonist, the effect on endothelial permeability is completely abolished, suggesting that local accumulation of bradykinin induced by this angiotensin converting enzyme inhibitor is responsible for the observed phenomenon. However, combined administration of captopril and R-705, a bradykinin-B1 receptor antagonist, fails to prevent the effects of this converting enzyme inhibitor. Intravenous injection of the bradykinin B1-receptor antagonist alone has no effect on endothelial permeability to Evans blue in the normal rat, whereas bradykinin alone is associated with a marked elevation in Evans blue extravasation in the pancreas, heart and duodenum [45].

Similar experiments performed in the SHR also revealed interesting results with captopril and perindopril [46]. In the untreated eight-weeks old SHR, there is a significant elevation in Evans blue extravasation in the following microcirculation networks: lung parenchyma, kidney, liver, pancreas, duode-

num, skin, and skeletal muscle. There are no changes in the heart and spleen microcirculation, whereas a significant decrement is observed in the trachea. The effect of angiotensin converting enzyme inhibition is illustrated in Figure 7. In the experiments reported, the drugs were administered by gavage in two groups of eight-week old SHR, over ten consecutive days. Captopril normalized Evans blue extravasation only in the lung parenchyma, kidney, liver and skleletal muscle, whereas perindopril reduced to baseline, and even slightly below baseline values, Evans blue leakage in all microcirculation networks examined. It is important to note that the reduction in blood pressure was comparable in the two groups of hypertensive animals, suggesting, therefore, that the effect of the two drugs on endothelial permeability was not related to the reduction in blood pressure. In a separate group of experiments, the effect of angiotensin AT1–receptor blockade with losartan was similarly studied in the SHR. In contrast to observations made with captopril and perindopril, losartan failed to normalize endothelial dysfunction associated with hypertension in most tissues examined. Only in the skeletal muscle microcirculation network was losartan effective. The mechanisms responsible for the differences observed with angiotensin converting enzyme inhibition and angiotensin AT1-receptor blockade are not readily apparent but could well be related with the non-angiotensin-dependent pharmacological effects of the former class of antihypertensive drugs, at least with regard to the endothelial permeability to albumin function in the microcirculation networks examined.

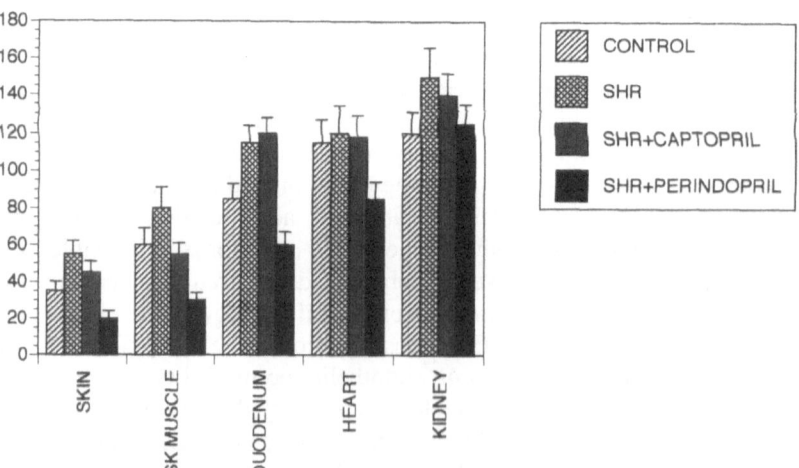

Figure 7. The effect of angiotensin converting enzyme inhibition on capillary permeability to Evans blue in spontaneously hypertensive rats was examined following ten days of therapy by gavage (modified from [46]).

ACE inhibition in the thoracic aorta vasa vasorum system

The microcirculation network of large blood vessels, namely the *vasa vasorum*, has been poorly studied, yet a potential role for this highly specialized microcirculation system in distribution arteries such as the aorta in the development of disease processes, including atherosclerosis and aneurysm is more than likely [47]. The regulation of blood flow in the *vasa vasorum* is still debated, particularly the capacity of these vessels to autoregulate; quite an important phenomenon, knowing that two-thirds of the aortic wall is perfused from the adventicial *vasa vasorum* [48]. In addition, according to some authors, this microcirculation network is involved in the clearance of macromolecules which penetrate from the lumen endothelial layer, including lipoproteins and cholesterol [49]. Only in recent studies have receptors for potent vaso-active mediators been identified in isolated *vasa vasorum* dissected from bovine aortic specimens [50–52].

Our interest in this field of research began from the first observation made on the consequences of disease processes, such as arterial hypertension and diabetes mellitus, on Evans blue extravasation in the aortic wall of experimental animals, and the effect of antihypertensive drugs on this unique phenomenon, not knowing in addition, from which side of the wall Evans blue was penetrating, the luminal or antiluminal [53]. As shown in Figure 8, the baseline

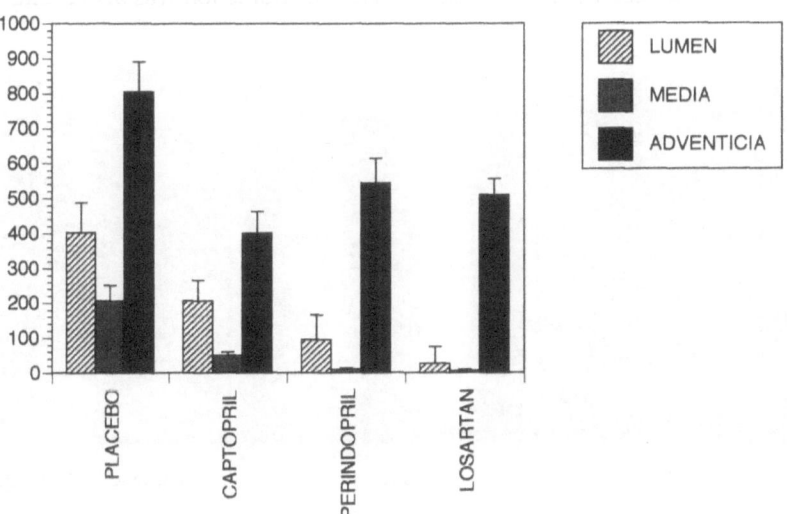

Figure 8. The effect of two angiotensin converting enzyme inhibitors and of losartan, an AT1 angiotensin receptor antagonist, on evans blue extravasation in normotensive and spontaneously hypertensive rats was examined. Drug treatment lasted ten days as in experiments shown in Figure 7 (modified from [53, 54]).

extravasation of Evans blue measured in the normal unanesthetized rat is relatively high (75 µg/mg dry weight), as much as 50% of Evans blue extravasation measured in the kidney, the most highly perfused organ. In the untreated SHR, Evans blue leakage is enhanced by approximately 30% above normal values in the thoracic and abdominal segments of the same vessel. In addition, the effect of two angiotensin converting enzyme inhibitors on this abnormality differ not only in potency, but also on anatomical selectivity: none of the drugs affect the abdominal segment of the aorta. Using fluorescence microscopy, where the blue color turns red, it became possible to localize the site of Evans blue penetration into the aortic wall. As illustrated in Figure 9, it is evident that much more Evans blue penetrates from the adventicia than from the lumimal endothelium [54]. The phenomenon is markedly enhanced, and from both sides of the aortic wall, in the untreated SHR. Again, partial correction of the endothelial dysfunction is different with captopril and perindopril, suggesting involvement of angiotensin- and/or bradykinin-dependent-phenomena degradation, as well as differences in the response to converting enzyme inhibition.

In order to study specifically the *vasa vasorum* micorcirculation system, an *in vitro* thoracic aorta perfusion model was developed to look at the arteriolar contractile activity, as well as the profile of endothelial permeability to Evans blue, in specimens obtained from normal rabbits. The characteristics of angiotensin-II AT1 and AT2 receptors and bradykinin B1 and B2 receptors were identified with the use of specific agonists and antagonists. As shown in Figure 10, the vasocontractile AT1-dependent action of angiotensin-II was identified in a dose-dependent fashion. This phenomenon was also found to be

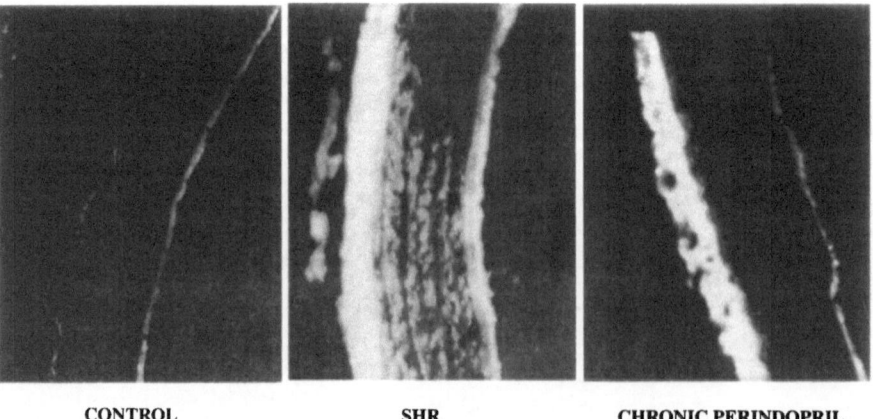

CONTROL   SHR   CHRONIC PERINDOPRIL

Figure 9. Regional distribution of Evans blue within the aortic wall obtained from representative control, untreated spontaneously hypertensive rat and spontaneously hypertensive rat treated with perindopril. The pictures examined by fluorescence microcopy clearly show the heterogeneous distribution of Evans blue in the luminal (right side) and antiluminal (left side) sides of the aortic wall (reproduced with permission from [54]).

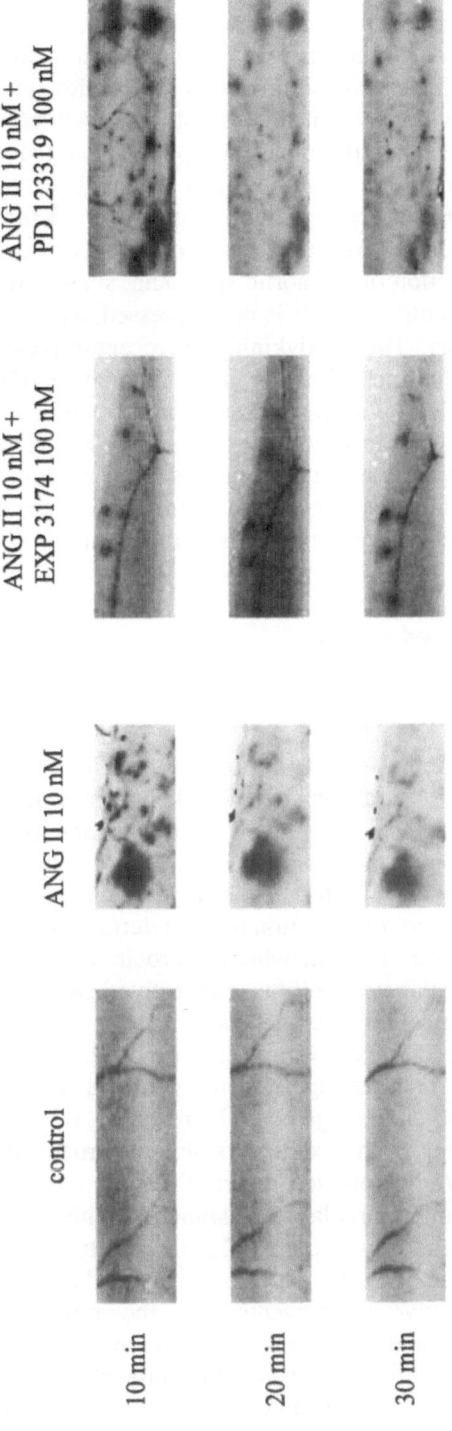

Figure 10. The contractile response of *vasa vasorum* arterioles, and the number of Evans blue extravasation spots from the microcirculation, before and following angiotensin administration is shown in this representative experiment performed *in vitro* on a segment of thoracic aorta obtained from a normal rabbit.

accompanied by a marked reduction in the number of extravasation spots measured on the outside surface of the aorta. AT1 receptor blockade abolished both vascular phenomena. Angiotensin-II was also associated with late arteriolar dilatation and Evans blue extravasation due to nitric oxide release via AT2 receptor stimulation, since blockade of this receptor, as well as inhibition of nitric oxide synthase, neutralized these vascular phenomena [51]. In another series of experiments, arteriolar dilatation and Evans blue extravasation induced by bradykinin B2 receptor stimulation were documented. The bradykinin B1 receptor-induced arteriolar vasocontriction was only apparent four hours following dissection of the aortic specimen, suggesting that under baseline control conditions this receptor is not expressed, as demonstrated in other vascular preparations. The bradykinin B1 receptor pharmacological actions become evident with time, following micro-traumatism of the vascular tissue [52]. These results clearly indicate that the thoracic aorta *vasa vasorum* microcirculation network is provided with the two angiotensin-II receptors and the bradykinin B2 receptor under normal conditions. The bradykinin B1 receptor is expressed under pathophysiological situations. Therefore, these receptors become potential targets for pharmacological interventions.

ACE inhibition in health and disease

Introduction

Most experimental and clinical studies reported on ACE inhibition in the microcirculation deal with arterial hypertension. It becomes more and more evident that the renin-angiotensin system and the non-angiotensin-II-dependent effects of ACE inhibition on the microvasculature play an important role in physiological conditions such as internal distribution of fluid and solutes, adaptation to environment, and mobilization of fluid during diuretic therapy or hemofiltration. Other disease states in which microcirculatory disturbances have been studied include diabetes mellitus, congestive heart failure, chronic renal insufficiency, vasculitis, and atherogenesis.

The importance of microcirculation in disease processes mainly relates to its potential role in target organ damage. Often regarded as a specific feature of a given disease, target organ damage could be regarded, on the contrary, as a non-specific event resulting from a pathophysiological process common to a variety of apparently different etiologies, a sort of common denominator. It is tempting to propose that microcirculation dysfunction, either in pre- and/or post-capillary resistances, and/or in endothelial permeability, is responsible for target organ damage. In fact, plasma extravasation into the interstitial compartment is associated with two major events. First, the volume of this strategic compartment increases, and depending on its initial size and it will augment the distance between blood flow and the intracellular compartment. Second, the interstitial composition changes because of fluid, small solutes, and macromolecule accumulation, especially if poor lymphatic drainage coexists. These features will affect the hydraulic coefficient and the albumin-exclusion phenomenon. As a consequence of these events, the traffic of vital substrates from blood to any cell mass, and removal of waste products in the opposite direction, will be affected; together menacing cell integrity and viability in a totally non-specific manner. This original and simple way to look at pathophysiology has been documented in an indirect way, by few investigators, and recently in a direct manner, by measuring interstitial oxygen tension when skeletal muscle blood flow is interrupted and the interstitial compartment rendered edematous [41].

Diabetes mellitus

Diabetes mellitus, a mostly serious metabolic disease which involves carbohydrate and lipid abnormalities, affects both the macro- and microcirculation. It is likely that the macrocirculation complications encountered in diabetes mellitus, such as accelerated atherogenesis, are related to microcirculatory defects in the *vasa vasorum* system, raising again the critical importance of this specialized network. Images of the latter network in thoracic aorta specimens obtained from alloxan-induced diabetes in the rabbit, show important arteriolar dilatation and massive Evans blue leakage [47]. In most other microcirculation networks, such as the heart, kidney, skeletal muscle, skin, and intestinal tract endothelial dysfunction characterized by enhanced permeability to albumin has been described [55, 56] and found to be bradykinin B1 receptor-mediated [56]. Microalbuminuria, a marker of the renal glomerular microcirculation dysfunction, has been successfully targeted by ACE inhibitors. It now appears that reduction of microalbuminuria is correlated with a significant reduction in the progression of glomerular insufficiency, a major achievement in the protection of this target organ in diabetes [57].

Nailfold capillaroscopy is becoming a new and elegant non-invasive approach to clinical microcirculation evaluation in diabetic patients. This approach even appears to be more sensitive than microalbuminuria screening to detect early endothelial dysfunction in diabetes mellitus. In a recent study performed in insulin-dependent diabetic patients showing no evidence of conventional vascular complications, including microalbuminuria, ACE inhibition with low-dose ramipril or captopril was associated with normalization of post-occlusive hyperemia abnormalities, as measured by nailfold capillaroscopy [58].

Congestive heart failure

Heart failure is becoming a major problem, not only because of its increasing incidence in elderly populations, but also because invasive cardiology is augmenting the longevity of a diseased organ. Conventional mono-therapy with diuretics has not overcome the problem of refractory edematous states. It is obvious that microcirculatory disturbances are responsible for resistance to diuretic therapy. In fact, most diuretic agents enhance capillary permeability to albumin and favor much more fluid and solute movements from the vascular to the interstitial compartments, which may temporarily relieve the stress imposed on both the left and right ventricles [59]. However, when solely administered in the congestive heart failure patient, these drugs represent a real handicap to fluid mobilization in the opposite direction, that is, from interstitial compartments back to the circulation, to be excreted by the kidneys.

ACE inhibition provides similar relief on both ventricles by decreasing peripheral resistance due to angiotensin-dependent effects [60] and likely also by bradykinin-dependent actions on microcirculation networks. In particular by increasing endothelial permeability, moving, like diuretics, fluid and solutes out of the vascular compartment. Using the local washout isotope method in two major fluid reservoirs, skeletal muscle and skin of the lower leg, Galatius et al. recently demonstrated in congestive heart failure patients, that ACE inhibition with fosinopril administered over 12 weeks, reduces vascular resistance in these two microcirculation networks much more in the muscle than in the skin [61].

It appears clear, therefore, that the problem encountered in congestive heart failure is not only a problem of transient stress relief on the left and right ventricles by pushing fluid out of the vascular space, but also of mobilizing accumulated fluid in the extravascular space (interstitial and intracellular) for renal excretion once the cardiac function is restored by positive inotropic treatment. The recent development of omapatrilat, a drug capable of simultaneous inhibition of angiotensin converting enzyme and neutral endopeptidase, may help in resolving the above-mentioned dilemma [62]. Since neutral endopeptidase is responsible for the degradation of natriuretic peptides, blocking this protease should prolong the half-life of peptides capable of increasing fluid and sodium excretion by the kidney in congestive heart failure patients. Preliminary clinical data obtained with this new drug are encouraging in this regard. However, pending questions will require additional experimental work with omapatrilat, such as potential bradykinin B1 receptor-mediated effects due to accumulation of desArg9-bradykinin [63], as well as the endothelial permeabilizing actions of natriuretic peptides in microcirculation networks [64]. Nevertheless, the emergence of this new class of drugs to be used in arterial hypertension and heart failure deserves admiration and hope for the new millennium [65].

References

1 Ganong WF (1997) Dynamics of blood and lymph flow. *In*: WF Ganong (ed.): *Review of Medical Physiology*. Appleton and Lange, Stamford, 536–552
2 Reed RK, Laurent UBG (1992) Turnover of hyaluronan in the microcirculation. *Amer Rev Respir*

Dis 146: S37–S39

3 Kiani MF, Pries AR, Hsu LL, Sarelius IH, Cokelet GR (1994) Fluctuations of microvascular blood flow parameters caused by hemodynamic mechanisms. *Amer J Physiol* 266: H1822–1828

4 Davies PF (1995) Flow-mediated endothelial mechanotransduction. *Physiol Rev* 75: 519–604

5 Simionescu N (1983) Cellular aspects of transcapillary exchange. *Physiol Rev* 63: 1536–1640

6 Soulis-Liparota T, Cooper M, Papazoglou D, Clarke B, Jerums G (1991) Retardation by aminoguanidine of developement of albuminuria, mesangial expansion and tissue fluorescence in streptozotocin-induced diabetic rat. *Diabetes* 40: 1328–1334

7 Chakir M, Plante GE (1996) Endothelial cell dysfunction in diabetes mellitus. *Prostagland Leukotriene Essent Fatty Acid* 54: 45–51

8 Click RL, Gilmore JP, Joyner WL (1977) Direct demonstration of alterations in the microcirculation of the hamster during and following renal hypertension. *Circ Res* 41: 461–467

9 Bohlen HG (1983) Intestinal microvascular adaptation during maturation of spontaneously hypertensive rats. *Hypertension* 5: 739–745

10 Engelson ET, Schmid-Sconbein GW, Zweifach BW (1986) The microvasculature in skeletal muscle: II. Arteriolar network anatomy in normotensive and spontaneously hypertensive rats. *Microvasc Res* 31: 356–374

11 Blantz RC, Konnen KS, Tucker BJ (1976) Angiotensin-II effects upon glomerular microcirculation and ultrafiltration coefficient of the rat. *J Clin Invest* 57: 419–434

12 Bohlen HG (1989) The microcirculation in hypertension. *J Hypertension* 7 (suppl 4): S117–S124

13 Lehoux S, Plante GE, Sirois MG, Sirois P, D'Orléans-Juste P (1992) Phosphoramidon blocks big-endothelin-1 but not endothelin-1 enhancement of vascular permeability in the rat. *Brit J Pharmacol* 107: 996–1000

14 Patterson CE, Rhoades RA, Garcia JGN (1992) Evans blue dye as a marker of albumin clearance in cultured endothelial monolayer and isolated lung. *J Appl Physiol* 72: 865–873

15 Lortie M, Gauthier B, Plante GE (1992) Renal reperfusion injury: sequential changes in function and regional albumin extravasation. *Microvasc Res* 48: 295–302

16 Plante GE, Dion D, Labrecque G (2001) Seasonal variations in endothelial permeability to albumin in the normal rat. *Can J Physiol Pharmacol*; *in press*

17 Larouche A, Lehoux S, Cadieux A, Sirois P, Plante GE (1998) Perméabilité endothéliale à l'albumine de la paroi aortique. *Médecine Sci* 14 (suppl 1): 23

18 Jung F, Wappler M, Nüttgens HP, Kiesewetter H, Wolf S, Müller G (1987) Video capillary microscopy: determination of geometrical and dynamic parameters. *Biomed Tech* 32: 204–213

19 Greene AS (1998) Life and death in the microcirculation: a role for angiotensin-II. Microcirculation 5: 101–107

20 Li JS, Schiffrin EL (1996) Effect of calcium channel blockade or angiotensin-converting enzyme inhibition on structure of coronary, renal, and other small arteries in spontaneously hypertensive rats. *J Cardiovasc Pharmacol* 28: 68–74

21 Scotland R, Vallance P, Ahluwalia A (1999) Endothelin alters the reactivity of vasa vasorum: mechanisms and implications for conduit vessel physiology and pathophysiology. *Brit J Pharmacol* 128: 1229–1234

22 Shao XP, Chainey A, Plante GE (2000) Pharmacologie des récepteurs de l'angiotensine-II dans la microcirculation de l'aorte thoracique. *Médecine Sci* 16: 12

23 Rene P, Simonson MS, Dunn MJ (1989) Physiology of the mesangial cell. *Physiol Rev* 69: 1347–1401

24 Sorbi D, Fadly M, Hicks R, Alexander S, Arbeit L (1993) Captopril inhibits the 72 kDa and 92 kDa matrix metalloproteinases. *Kidney Int* 44: 1266–1272

25 Simon G, Altman S (1992) Subpressor angiotensin II is a bifunctional growth factor of vascular muscle in rats. *J Hypertension* 10: 1165–1171

26 Bussien JP, d'Amore TF, Perret L (1986) Single and repeated dosing of the converting enzyme inhibitor perindopril to normal subjects. *Clin Pharmacol Ther* 39: 554–558

27 Unger T, Moursi M, Ganten D, Hermann K, Lang RE (1986) Antihypertensive action of the converting enzyme inhibitor perindopril (S9490-3) in spontaneously hypertensive rat: comparison with enalapril (MK421) and ramipril (HOE498). *J Cardiovasc Pharmacol* 8: 276–285

28 Vacek L, Braveny P (1978) Effect of angiotensin-II on blood pressure and microvascular beds in mesentery, skin, and skeletal muscle of the rat. *Microvasc Res* 16: 43–50

29 Meininger GA, Harris PD, Joshua IG (1984) Distributions of microvascular pressure in skeletal muscle of one-kidney, one-clip, two-kidney, one-clip and deoxycorticosterone-salt hypertensive

rats. *Hypertension* 6: 27–34

30 Bohlen HG (1989) The microcirculation in hypertension. *J Hypertension* 7 (suppl 4): S117–S124

31 Myers TO, Joyner WL, Gilmore FP (1988) Angiotensin reactivity in the cheek pouch of the renovascular hypertensive hamster. *Hypertension* 12: 373–379

32 Vicaut E, Hou X (1993) Arteriolar constriction and local renin-angiotensin In rat microcirculation. *Hypertension* 21: 491–497

33 Mohama RE, Joyner WL, Gilmore JP (1984) Comparative reactivity of hamster cheek pouch microvessels to arginine vasopressin and angiotensin II. *Microcirc Endothel Lymphat* 1: 397–413

34 Hutchins PM, Darnell AE (1974) Observation of a decrease in number of small arterioles in spontaneously hypertensive rat. *Circ Res* 34/35 (suppl 1): 161–165

35 Le Noble J, Tangelder GJ, Slaff DW, VanEssen H, Reneman RS, Struyker-Boudier HAJ (1990) A functional morphometric study of the cremaster muscle microcirculation in young spontaneously hypertensive rats. *J Hypertension* 8: 741–748

36 Bohlen HG (1979)Arteriolar closure mediated by hyperresponsiveness to norepinephrine in hypertensive rats. *Amer J Physiol* 236: H157–H164

37 Hashimoto H, Prewitt RL, Efaw CW (1987) Alterations in the microvasculature of one-kidney, one-clip hypertensive rats. *Amer J Physiol* 253: H933–H940

38 Hernandez I, Cowley AW, Lombard JH, Greene AS (1992) Salt intake and angiotensin II alter microvessel density in the cremaster muscle of normal rats. *Amer J Physiol* 263: H664–H667

39 Plante GE, Bissonnette M, Sirois MG, Regoli D, Sirois P (1992) Renal permeability alteration precedes hypertension and involves bradykinin in the spontaneously hypertensive rat. *J Clin Invest* 89: 2030–2034

40 Comper WD, Laurent TC (1978) Physiological function of connective tissue polysaccharides. *Physiol Rev* 58: 255–315

41 Plante GE, Chakir M, Lehoux S, Lortie M (1995) Disorders of body fluid balance: a new look into the mechanisms of disease. *Can J Cardiol* 11: 788–802

42 Gottlieb AI, Langile BL, Wong MK, Kim DW (1991) Structure and function of the endothelial cytoskeleton. *Lab Invest* 65: 123–137

43 Lehoux S, Plante GE (2001) Key role of cytoskeletal and extracellular matrix proteins in the maintenance of capillary barrier function *in vivo*. *Circ Res*; *in press*

44 Lehoux S, Plante GE (1994) Contrasting effects of various antihypertensives on capillary permeability in the normal rat. *J Amer Soc Nephrol* 5: 348

45 Lehoux S, Plante GE (1996) Antihypertensive drugs and endothelial cell function. *Prostagland Leukotriene Essent Fatty Acid* 54: 65–70

46 Lehoux S, Plante GE (2001) Heterogeneity of capillary permeability response to antihypertensive drug regimens in the spontaneously hypertensive rat. *Microvasc Res*; *in press*

47 Plante GE, Alfred J, Chakir M (1999) The blood vessel, linchpin of diabetic lesions. *Metabolism* 48: 406–409

48 Heistad DD, Marcus ML, Law EG, Armstrong ML, Ehrhardy JC, Abhoud FM (1978) Regulation of blood flow to the aortic media in dogs. *J Clin Invest* 62: 133–139

49 Bemin J, Corman B, Merval R, Tedgui A (1993) Age-related changes in endothelial permeability and distribution volume of albumin in rat aorta. *Amer J Physiol* 264: H679–H685

50 Scotland R, Vallance P, Ahluwalia A (1999) Endothelin alters the reactivity of vasa vasorum: mechanisms and implications for conduit vessel physiology and pathophysiology. *Brit J Pharmacol* 128: 1229–1234

51 Shao X, Chainey A, Plante GE (2001) Pharmacologie des récepteurs de l'angiotensine-II dans la microcirculation de l'aorte thoracique. *Médecine Sci* 16 (suppl 1): 34

52 Shao X, Chainey A, Plante GE (2001) Bradykinin B1 and B2 receptor-mediated vaso-active effects in vasa vasorum of rabbit thoracic aorta *in vitro*. *Brit J Pharmacol*; *in press*

53 Lehoux S, Larouche A, Cadieux A, Plante GE (1995) Perméabilité endothéliale de l'aorte du rat spontanément hypertendu: effets de divers antihypertenseurs. *Arch Mal Cœur Vaisseaux* 88: 62

54 Plante GE, Lehoux S, Larouche A, Brière N, Cadieux A (2001) Antihypertensive agents affect endothelial function in the thoracic aorta: pathophysiological significance. *Can J Physiol Pharmacol*; *in press*

55 Tooke JE (1995) Microvascular function in human diabetes: a physiological perspective. *Diabetes* 44: 721–726

56 Chakir M, Plante GE (1996) Endothelial cell dysfunction in diabetes mellitus. *Prostagland Leukotriene Essent Fatty Acid* 54: 45–51

57 Mathiesen ER, Hommel E, Hansen HP (1997) Preservation of normal GFR with long-term captopril treatment in normotensive IDDM patients with microalbuminuria. *J Amer Soc Nephrol* 8: 115A

58 Haak E, Haak T, Kusterer K, Reschke B, Faust H, Usadel KH (1998) Microcirculation in hyperglycemic patients with IDDM without diabetic complications-effect of low-dose angiotensin-converting enzyme inhibition. *Exp Clin Endocrinol Diabetes* 106: 45–50

59 Lehoux S, Sirois MG, Sirois P, Plante GE (1994) Acute and chronic diuretic treatment selectively affects vascular permeability in the unanesthetized normal rat. *J Pharmacol Exp Ther* 269: 1094–1099

60 Harris P (1987) Congestive heart failure: central role of the arterial blood pressure. *Brit Heart J* 59: 190–203

61 Galatius S, Wroblewski H, Sorensen V, Haunso S, Norgaard T, Kastrup J (1999) Reversal of peripheral microvascular dysfunction during long-term treatment with the angiotensin-converting enzyme inhibitor fosinopril in congestive heart failure. *J Cardiac Fail* 5: 17–24

62 Burnett JC (1999) Vasopeptidase inhibition: a new concept in blood pressure management. *J Hypertension* 17: S37–S43

63 Décarie A, Raymond P, Gervais N, Couture R, Adam A (1996) Serum interspecies differences in metabolic pathways of bradykinin and [desArg9]BK: influence of enalaprilat. *Amer J Physiol* 270: H1340–H1347

64 Espiner EA (1994) Physiology of natriuretic peptides. *J Int Med* 235: 527–541

65 Plante GE (2000) Traitement sans bogue de l'hypertension artérielle au nouveau millénaire. Nouvelle pharmacologie du système rénine angiotensine. *Médecine Sci* 16 (suppl 1): 14–17

ACE Inhibitors
ed. by P. D'Orléans-Juste and G.E. Plante
© 2001 Birkhäuser Verlag/Switzerland

Arterial structure and function and blockade of the renin-angiotensin system in hypertension

Michel E. Safar[1], Harry A.J. Struijker Boudier[2], Luc M.A.B. Van Bortel[2] and Gérard M. London[3]

[1] *Department of Internal Medicine, Broussais Hospital, F-75674-Paris, France*
[2] *Department of Pharmacology, University of Limburg, 6200 MD -Maastricht, The Netherlands*
[3] *Service de Néphrologie, Centre Hospitalier F.H. Manhes, F-91700-Fleury Mérogis, France*

Introduction

Cardiovascular disease is a major cause of morbidity and mortality in patients with hypertension. Epidemiological and clinical studies have shown that damage of large conduit arteries is a major contributory factor [1]. Macrovascular disease develops slowly in hypertensive patients and is responsible for the high incidence of congestive heart failure, left ventricular hypertrophy (LVH), ischemic heart disease, sudden death, cerebrovascular accidents and peripheral artery diseases. Although the most frequent underlying cause of these complications is occlusive lesions due to atheromatous plaques, this aspect represents only one form of the structural response to metabolic and hemodynamic alterations which interfere with the hypertensive process. The spectrum of arterial alterations in hypertension is broader, including large artery hypertrophy associated with hemodynamic burden [2]. The consequences of these alterations may be different from those attributed to the presence of atherosclerotic plaques alone. In this chapter, the basic concepts on changes in arterial structure and function in hypertension are reviewed and their alterations in response to the blockade of the renin-angiotensin system are discussed in experimental and clinical situations.

Basic concepts

Mechanical factors acting on the arterial wall: an overview

The arterial wall is a complex tissue composed of different cell populations capable of structural and functional changes in response to direct injury and atherogenic factors or to changes in long-term hemodynamic conditions [3]. The principal geometric modifications induced by hemodynamic alterations are changes in the width of the arterial lumen and/or arterial wall thickness [4] due to activation, proliferation and migration of smooth muscle cells and rearrangements of cellular elements and extracellular matrix of the vessel wall [3].

The mechanical signals for changes of arterial structure associated with hemodynamic overload are the cyclic tensile stress and/or shear stress [3–5]. Blood pressure is the principal determinant of arterial wall stretch and tensile stress, creating radial and tangential forces that counteract the effect of intraluminal pressure. Blood flow alterations result in changes of shear stress – the dragging frictional force created by blood flow. While acute changes in tensile or shear stress induce transient adjustments in arterial diameter, chronic alterations in mechanical forces lead to changes in the geometry and composition of the vessel wall that may be considered adaptive responses to long lasting changes in blood flow and/or pressure [1, 4–6].

According to Laplace's law, tensile stress (s) is directly proportional to arterial transmural pressure (P) and radius (r), and inversely proportional to arterial wall thickness (h) according to the formula: $s = Pr/h$. In response to increased blood pressure or arterial radius, tensile stress is maintained within the physiological range by thickening of the vessel wall.

Shear stress is a function of the blood flow pattern [3–6]. In "linear" segments of the vasculature, blood is displaced in layers moving at different velocities. The middle of the stream moves more rapidly than the side layers, generating the parabolic velocity profile. The slope of the velocity profile, i.e., the change in blood velocity per unit distance across the vessel radius, defines the shear rate. Shear stress is the product of shear rate times blood viscosity. Shear stress (t) is directly proportional to blood flow (Q) and blood viscosity (μ) and inversely proportional to the radius (r) of the vessel, according to the formula: $t = 4Q\mu/r^3$. Increased shear stress could be the consequence of increased blood viscosity, decreased arterial diameter or increased blood flow and blood flow gradient applied to the vessel-blood interface. Changes of shear and tensile stresses are interrelated, because any modification of arterial radius caused by alterations of blood flow and shear stress induces changes of tensile stress (unless the pressure varies in the opposite direction).

The process of transmission of mechanical forces from the blood to the cells and force transduction within the cells are incompletely understood. Detailed descriptions of the mechanisms of mechanotransduction and the biology of the remodeling are beyond the scope of this chapter and are available elsewhere [7, 8]. The process of transforming mechanical forces into rearrangement of the vascular system implies that there are "sensors" that detect and transmit physical forces to effector cells. Endothelial cells are strategically situated at the blood vessel wall interface and are the principal candidates for the role of "sensors" [7, 8]. Endothelial cells are principally involved in sensing and transducing shear stress, and the candidate mechanosensors are integrin-matrix-cytoskeleton interaction, mechanosensitive K^+-ion channels, G proteins, and caveolae [7]. This mechanosensor activation results in the transduction of physical stimuli into a biochemical signal affecting arterial function through the generation of nitric oxide, prostacyclin, endothelium-derived hyperpolarizing factor, endothelins, adhesion molecule expression, and activation of thrombotic and antithrombotic factors [9]. Endothelial cells also participate in vascular structure by releasing and/or activating growth factors, like platelet-derived growth factor, fibroblast growth factor, transforming growth factor- and extracellular matrix regulators, influencing the growth, migration, phenotype and apoptosis of vascular smooth muscle cells [9, 10]. While shear stress acts mainly on endothelial cells, changes in tensile stress are sensed by the entire vessel wall and vascular smooth muscle cells respond directly to changes in cyclic stretch which seems essential for the maintenance of the contractile phenotype [4, 6, 11].

Hypertension and large artery structure

The characteristics of arterial structure depend largely on the nature of hemodynamic stimuli applied to the vessel [12, 13]. To maintain tensile stress within physiological limits, arteries respond by thickening their walls (Laplace's law). The increased tensile stress is due to the direct effect of high pressure and the pressure-dependent passive distension of the arterial lumen [2]. *In vivo* studies on animals and humans have shown that this passive pressure-dependent distension of the arterial diameter is limited in the case of central (elastic type) arteries, and even absent for peripheral (muscular type) arteries, thus causing an increase of the wall to lumen ratio which is proportional to the blood pressure level [3, 14]. The limited or absent pressure-dependent increase in diameter efficiently maintains tensile stress within normal ranges, resulting in arterial hypertrophy and, in some cases, in remodeling [15]. Because, for a given pressure, the r/h ratio must remain constant, this unchanged ratio is obviously maintained through a wide range of r- and h-values, a situation which implies a major role for non-hemodynamic mechanisms [10]. Although the detailed analysis of such alterations is beyond the scope of this review, two main findings are stressed in this contribution. First, arterial structure is tightly modulated by environmental factors, such as the dietary sodium intake and ovarian hormones [16, 17]. Experimental studies have shown that increased sodium intake and absence of oestrogens are associated with increased arterial wall thickness and extracellular matrix, independently of blood pressure changes. In contrast, sodium restriction, use of diuretics and presence of oestrogens are associated with a smaller wall thickness and extracellular matrix [16, 17]. The second point to consider is that, among the numerous well-known growth or antigrowth factors acting on the arterial wall, antihypertensive compounds acting on the renin-angiotensin system have a major influence.

In recent years, several arguments have suggested that angiotensin II acts not only on arterioles but also on arteries [18, 19]. Angiotensin II (Ang II) receptors are widely distributed throughout the vascular tree from resistance arterioles to the aorta. Ang II produces contractions in aortic strips or rings as well as in isolated femoral, carotid, and coronary arteries. Moreover, Ang II seems to alter the arterial wall in hypertension by mechanisms other than the increase in blood pressure [20–23]: (i) components of the renin-angiotensin system are present within the endothelium and the arterial wall, a specific site where Ang II generation has been demonstrated [24, 25]; (ii) Ang II induces arterial hypertrophy and, moreover, a significant collagen production in vascular smooth muscle cell cultures [26–29]; (iii) *in vivo* administration of non-pressor doses of Ang II produces arterial thickening [29, 30]. Along this latter line of evidence, it has been possible using angiotensin-converting enzyme (ACE) inhibitors and Ang II antagonists, to obtain regression or prevention of structural arterial alterations in animal hypertension. Some observations are even consistent with the possibility that converting enzyme inhibitors have specific effects on the structure independently of their antihypertensive action. During ACE inhibition, not only the inhibition of Ang II, but also other factors such as bradykinin activation, attenuation of the sympathetic nervous system, and changes in endothelial function might also influence the vascular structure.

Arterial wall and endothelial function

Experimental and clinical data indicate that acute and chronic augmentations of the arterial blood flow induce proportional increases in the vessel lumen, whereas decreasing the flow reduces arterial inner diameter [31, 32]. An example is the flow-mediated change in arterial structure associated with arterial dilation due to sustained high blood flow following the creation of an arteriovenous fistula [6]. In this situation, the lumen diameter increases to maintain shear stress within physiological limits. Increased arterial inner diameter is usually accompanied by arterial wall hypertrophy and increased intima media cross-sectional area (consecutive to increases in the radius and wall tension). The presence of the endothelium is a prerequisite for normal vascular adaptation to chronic changes in blood flow, and experimental data indicate that flow-mediated arterial remodeling could be decreased by inhibiting nitric oxide synthase [33]. Although the alterations in tensile and shear stresses are interrelated, changes in tensile stress primarily induce hypertrophy of the arterial media, whereas changes in shear stress principally modify the dimensions and structure of the intima [5, 7, 34]. This situation is particularly observed in the early phase of spontaneous hypertension in rats in which carotid artery diameter remains within the normal range despite the presence of high blood pressure and the presence of a transient increase in cardiac output and blood flow [35].

Experimental studies have also demonstrated an important role of the endothelium in the control of the viscoelastic properties of the arterial wall. Destruction of the endothelial layer of arteries experimentally subjected to physiological pressure induces an increase in the arterial diameter in parallel with an increase in compliance and a decrease in arterial wall viscosity [36,

37]. This finding suggests that an intact endothelium is necessary to maintain arterial diameter, compliance and distensibility within a physiologically acceptable range and that the effect of vasoconstrictive compounds, such as angiotensin II or norepinephrine, is involved in this process. Such agents are known to interact physiologically with NO and might contribute to maintain arterial geometry and function within a normal range [3, 10, 21].

Arterial functions

The arterial system has two distinct, interrelated hemodynamic functions [4]: 1) to deliver an adequate supply of blood from the heart to peripheral tissues, i.e., the *conduit function*; and 2) to dampen blood pressure oscillations caused by intermittent ventricular ejection, the *cushioning function*. These two aspects of arterial function are intricately interwoven but can be dealt with independently because they have different origins and consequences. Disorders of the conduit function result from the narrowing of the arterial lumen with ischemia affecting the tissues and organs downstream, while disorders of the cushioning function reflect alterations in arterial wall viscoelastic properties and have deleterious effects upstream on the heart and the arteries themselves.

Conduit function of arteries

The main function of arteries is to deliver at all times an adequate supply of blood to peripheral tissues and organs in accordance with their metabolic needs. Conduit function efficiency is the consequence of the width of the arteries and the very low resistance of large arteries to flow. Under normal conditions, the mean blood pressure is almost constant along the arterial tree (the mean blood pressure drops between the ascending aorta and arteries in the forearm or leg: about 2–3 mmHg in supine position) [38] and conduit function is primarily dependent on the diameter of the arterial lumen. The conduit function is highly efficient allowing an increase in cardiac output of 5–6-fold, thereby increasing the flow to some tissues, like muscles, perhaps 10-fold. This physiological adaptability is mediated through acute changes in arterial flow velocity and/or diameter. Diameter changes are dependent on the endothelium, which responds to alterations of shear stress [9, 39]. The acute endothelium-dependent vasodilatation is decreased in several clinical conditions, for example, atherosclerosis, hypertension, cardiac failure, hypercholesterolemia, diabetes, menopause and aging [3, 10].

Arterial structural changes associated with long-term pressure overload is characterized by a normal or slightly increased diameter of conduit arteries under baseline conditions and, therefore, with normal baseline conductive properties [40]. Under conditions of long-term flow overload, the arterial diameters are enlarged and baseline arterial conductance is increased [4, 41].

However, these chronic alterations are frequently accompanied by inadequate responses to an acute demand for a higher blood flow [4]. The principal long-term disturbance of conduit function occurs through narrowing or occlusion of arteries with restriction of blood flow and downstream ischemia or infarction of tissues. Atherosclerosis, characterized by the presence of plaques and arterial narrowing, is the most common occlusive vascular disease that disturbs conduit function. Atherosclerosis usually narrows an artery in an irregular fashion, with focal compensatory enlargement occurring at discrete sites of narrowing immediately adjacent to more-or-less normal areas [5]. Due to the large luminal area of conduit arteries, basal blood flow remains unchanged until the lumen diameter is narrowed by 50%. In this situation the capacity to acutely increase flow during activity is progressively impaired, but partially compensated by arteriolar vasodilation. Beyond a 70–80% reduction in the lumen diameter (critical stenosis), basal blood flow is reduced as is the ability to increase flow during activity [4].

Cushioning function of arteries

The main role of arteries as cushions is to dampen the pressure oscillations resulting from intermittent ventricular ejection ("Windkessel" effect) and to transform the pulsatile flow of arteries into the steady flow required in peripheral tissues and organs [4]. The large arteries can instantaneously accommodate the volume of blood ejected from the heart. Under normal conditions during systole, roughly 40% of stroke volume is forwarded directly to peripheral tissues, while the remainder is stored in capacitance arteries (mainly aorta and central arteries), distending the walls and storing the remaining 60% of stroke volume. About 10% of the energy produced by the heart is diverted for the distension of arteries and "stored" in the walls to be available during diastole. During diastole, most of the stored energy recoils the aorta, squeezing the stored blood forward into the peripheral tissues, thereby ensuring a continuous perfusion of organs and tissues. For the cushioning function to be efficient, the energy required for arterial distension and recoil should be as low as possible; in other words, for a given stroke volume, the pulse pressure should be as low as possible. The efficiency of the Windkessel function depends on the viscoelastic properties of arterial walls and the geometry of the arteries including their diameter and length [4]. The ability of arteries to instantaneously accommodate the volume ejected by the left ventricle can be described in terms of *compliance, distensibility* or *stiffness* of the aorta or an individual artery. These terms express the contained volume of the vasculature (total or segmental) as a function of a given transmural pressure over the physiological range of pressure. Compliance is a term that describes indirectly the absolute amount of change in strain following a change in stress. In physiology, compliance (C) is defined as the change in volume (V) due to a change in pressure (P), that is $C = V/P$. The reciprocal value of compliance is the elastance ($E = P/V$). Compliance represents the slope (delta V/delta P) of the pressure (P)–volume (V) relationship at a specific point on the pressure-volume curve. The arterial media is responsible for the vessel's physical properties. Because it is composed of a "mixture" of smooth muscle cells and connective tissue, containing elastin and collagen fibers, the pressure-volume relationship is nonlinear. At a low distending pressure, the tension is born by elastin fibers, whereas at a high distending pressure, the tension is predominantly borne by less extensible collagen fibers and the arterial wall becomes stiffer (less compliant) [4]. This arrangement is advantageous because it prevents arterial blood from pooling at high pressure and protects arteries from high pressure-induced rupture. To facilitate comparisons of viscoelastic properties of structures with different initial dimensions, compliance can be expressed relative to the initial volume as a coefficient of distensibility $D =$ delta V/delta $P \cdot V$, where delta V/delta P is compliance; V is here the initial volume. In contrast to distensibility or compliance which provides information about the "elasticity" of the artery as a hollow structure, the elastic incremental modulus (E_{inc}; Young's modulus) provides direct information, independently of vessel geometry, on the intrinsic elastic properties of the materials of the arterial wall. An increased E_{inc} is characteristic of stiffer biomaterials [4] and is responsible for the leftward shift of the pressure-volume curve. Arterial volume per unit length is equal to the arterial cross-sectional area, depending on arterial diameter (D). In that conditions, the definition of stiffness indices is simplified, D taking the place of V, and assuming a constant length of the artery. These different indexes are usually measured by ultrasound techniques which enable stroke changes of arterial diameters and arterial intima media thickness to be determined [2, 4, 42]. The stress applied to arterial segments (delta P) is the pulse pressure. Because of the nonhomogeneity of the viscoelastic properties of successive arterial segments and the effect of arterial wave reflections, pulse and systolic pressures are amplified from the aorta to the peripheral arteries and, in young and middle-aged subjects, brachial and peripheral pulse pressures overestimate the corresponding pressures in the aorta and central arteries [4]. To accurately determine the elastic properties of arterial segments, the "local" pulse pressure must be measured and taken into consideration. Pulse pressure can be assessed in central arteries like the aorta or carotid artery using applanation tonometry and a generalized transfer function [43, 44]. As an alternative technique to ultrasound, arterial distensibility can be evaluated by measuring the pulse wave velocity (PWV) over a given arterial segment [4, 45]. PWV increases with arterial stiffening [46]. The viscoelastic properties of arterial walls determine the amplitude of pressure waves as well as their propagation and reflections along the arterial tree [4, 47].

The cushioning function is altered by decreased distensibility and by stiffening of arterial walls. Major consequences of arterial stiffening are an increase in systolic and decrease in diastolic pressure with a high pulse pressure [4, 10]. Pulse pressure is an independent predictor of cardiovascular risk for the heart, particularly for the prediction of myocardial infarction [48–51].

Pulse pressure depends on the interaction between LV ejection (stroke volume and duration of systole) and the physical properties of the arterial system that influence pulse pressure by two mechanisms. The first, *direct mechanism*, involves the generation of a higher pressure wave by the LV ejecting into a stiff arterial system, and increased diastolic recoil resulting in a lower diastolic pressure. The second, *indirect* mechanism, acts via the influence of increased arterial stiffness on PWV and the timing of incident and reflected pressure waves [4, 47]. It is beyond the scope of the present chapter to provide a detailed description of the latter subject.

In hypertension, increased arterial stiffness appears largely to be caused by the elevated level of blood pressure as such, but there is increasing evidence that alterations in the arterial wall associated with hypertension also contribute to the changes in viscoelastic properties (see review in [2]). To elucidate this point, arterial compliance and distensibility should be compared at the same pressure in the normotensive and hypertensive population (isobaric compliance and distensibility) [4]. In animal models of hypertension, studies of arterial strips and rings indicate that isobaric compliance and distensibility are decreased, particularly in fully relaxed vessels [4, 52]. In human hypertension, for the same mean arterial pressure in the whole arterial tree, compliance and distensibility are decreased significantly in central arteries (aorta, carotid artery) [2, 4] but remain within the normal range in peripheral arteries (radial artery) [53]. The effect of hypertension on isobaric compliance differs markedly from one species to another and also from one vascular territory to another. Whereas in hypertensive men isobaric distensibility and compliance are normal for the radial [53] and common carotid arteries, they are decreased for the femoral artery [54]. In hypertensive rats, normal [53] as well as decreased [55] isobaric distensibility and compliance of the common carotid artery have been reported. For the thoracic aorta, which represents the major component of total arterial compliance, isobaric measurements have clearly shown decreased values in hypertensive rats [56] and humans [57]. These different patterns imply that the response of large artery to converting enzyme inhibition or AT_1 blockade may depend largely on the vascular territory studied.

Conduit arteries and blockade of the renin-angiotensin system

Experimental studies

Whereas in a majority of studies described in the literature, the stiffness of the arterial wall in hypertensive animals has been evaluated on strips or rings of vascular tissue [4, 52], recent investigations have been carried out on living dogs and rats [53–56]. *In vivo* studies using Doppler measurements of aortic wall movement have the advantage of providing dynamic data, but these data remain limited to the operational range of blood pressure of the corresponding animals. Furthermore, dynamic compliance is a complex parameter which is influenced not only by changes in smooth muscle tone and in structure of the arterial wall, but also by the frequency dependence of the elastic arterial modulus and by the viscosity of the arterial wall. For pharmacological studies, it is important to minimize the two latter factors in order to evaluate predominantly the drug-induced changes in arterial structure and smooth muscle tone. Thus, the determination of static compliance can offer additional information. In order to evaluate static compliance, *in situ* preparations using 18–20 mm of non-exposed common carotid artery have been developed to establish the compliance-pressure relationship over a wide range of transmural pressures from 0 to 200 mmHg (Fig. 1). Because the arterial tissue is heterogeneous [36, 55, 58] and involves both smooth muscle and extracellular matrix, the compliance-pressure relationship was found to be curvilinear [36, 55, 58], indicating that (i) within the lower transmural pressure ranges, in which tension is born by elastin and arterial smooth muscle tone, compliance increases strikingly with increasing pressure, whereas (ii) within the higher pressure ranges, tension is rather borne by collagen fibers, causing compliance to decrease with pressure.

Studies on *in situ* carotid artery preparations show that converting enzyme inhibition increases compliance independently of transmural pressure, when given either locally [36] or after acute oral administration [59]. The compli-

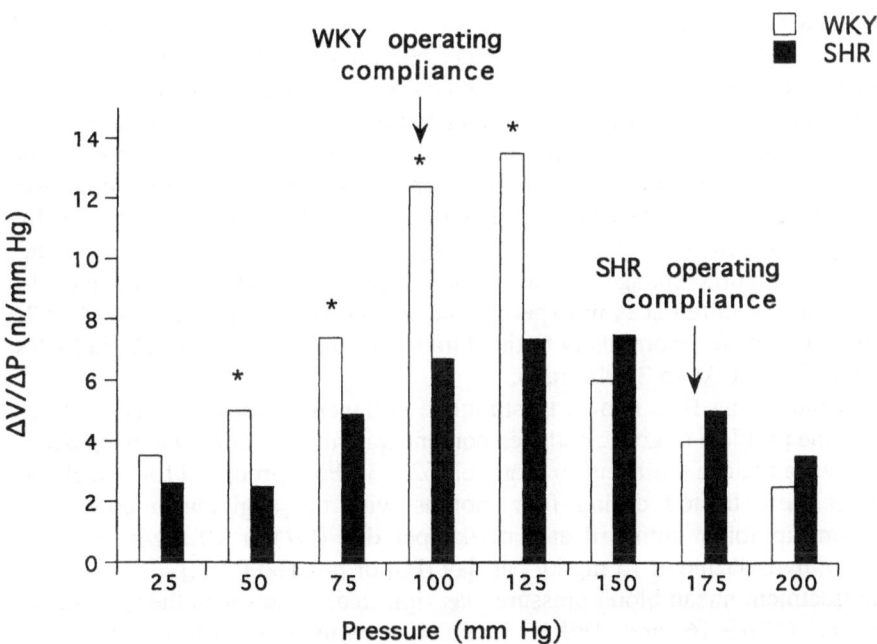

Figure 1. Carotid preparation: relationship between carotid compliance (ΔV/ΔP) and transmural pressure in normotensive (WKY) and hypertensive (SHRs) rats under baseline conditions [36, 55, 58]. *P < 0.001 (WKY *versus* SHRs). White bars represent WKY, black bars represent SHR rats. Data are mean. Δ represents delta (see text).

ance enhancement is obtained within the lower pressure ranges and disappears in the absence of endothelium, indicating that some of the effects of ACE inhibitors on the viscoelastic properties of the arterial wall may depend on endothelial function [36]. The same result is obtained using saralasin or bradykinin, instead of the converting enzyme inhibitor itself, but most studies suggest that the major role during the compliance increase is played by Ang II [60, 61]. The increase is observed even when the converting enzyme inhibitor given orally does not induce a significant reduction in systemic blood pressure [36, 59], suggesting that a decrease in arterial smooth muscle tone is associated with an improvement in the viscoelastic properties of the arterial wall.

In order to evaluate the structural changes associated with compliance modifications, the effects of chronic ACE inhibition on the function and the histomorphometric composition of the carotid artery and the aorta were studied in two-kidney, one-clip (2K-1C) Goldblatt hypertensive rats, in spontaneously hypertensive rats (SHRs) and compared with age-matched normotensive rats [36, 55, 58]. At the end of the treatment period, hemodynamic patterns were recorded and passive mechanical properties of the isolated carotid artery were measured *in situ*. Morphological parameters of the thoracic aortic wall, including media thickness, nucleus density, and elastin and collagen contents, were measured using an automated system. In the hypertensive models, hypertension was associated with a stiffer arterial wall, as demonstrated by an increase in characteristic impedance of the aorta, a decrease in systemic arterial compliance, and a decrease in carotid artery compliance. Chronic ACE inhibition normalized blood pressure and reversed these *in vivo* markers of vascular stiffness. The functional changes were obtained in parallel with structural modifications of the arterial wall. The increased aortic media thickness observed in hypertension was reversed. This reduction in the aortic media thickness was mainly related to a reduction in smooth muscle cell hypertrophy as assessed by a significant increase in nucleus density. There was no, or only a slight, decrease in aortic collagen content. The differential effects on collagen could be related to differences in experimental models, and/or to the dose of ACE inhibition, and/or more likely to the duration of treatment (12 weeks in SHRs *versus* four weeks in 2K-1C rats).

Because Ang II is known to stimulate collagen synthesis in cell cultures [28], the problem of aortic collagen content was further addressed using a preventive (and not a therapeutic) protocol [62, 63]. Four groups of four-week old SHRs were treated during four months with the angiotensin converting enzyme inhibitor quinapril at 1 mg/kg per day (Q1) or 10 mg/kg per day (Q10), hydralazine at 15 mg/kg per day (H), or placebo P [62]. At the end of the treatment, mean blood pressure was significantly lower in the Q10 and H groups (136 ± 16 and 149 ± 11 mmHg) compared with the P group (190 ± 23 mmHg) (Tab. 1). In the Q1 group there was only a slight reduction in mean blood pressure with values lower than the P group but significantly higher than the Q10 and H groups. The decrease in aortic medial cross-sectional area largely paralleled those of the blood pressure changes. In contrast,

Table 1. Prevention protocol in SHRs (see text): Histomorphometric parameters of thoracic aorta after four months of treatment [62]

	P (n = 12)	Q1 (n = 12)	Q10 (n = 12)	H (n = 12)
Media thickness (μm)	125 ± 19	115 ± 9	101 ± 12*†	99 ± 13*‡
Elastin content (× 10² μm²/mm)	29.1 ± 6.5	26.2 ± 4.9	23.8 ± 3.4	27.2 ± 4.1
Collagen density (%)	17.6 ± 3.9	12.7 ± 3.6*#	14.3 ± 4.1\\	18.8 ± 4.9
Collagen content (× 10² μm²/mm)	21.9 ± 4.7	15.3 ± 4.6*	14.3 ± 4.0*\\	18.6 ± 5.0
Nuclei density (No per field)	10.3 ± 1.8	14.6 ± 4.8¶	15.5 ± 3.6\\¶	19.7 ± 6.0*†
Nuclei content (per mm)	240 ± 58	292 ± 59	291 ± 87	322 ± 58

P indicates placebo; Q1, 1 mg/kg quinapril; Q10, 10 mg/kg quinapril; H, hydralazine. Values are mean ± SD; n is number of animals.
* p < 0.01, ¶ p < .05 vs P; ‡ p < .01; †p < .05 vs Q1; # p < .01; \\ p < .05 vs H.

in the Q10 and Q1 groups, the collagen content of the aortic media was significantly lower than in the two other groups and no difference was observed between Q1 and Q10 (Tab. 1). Aortic angiotensin converting enzyme activity was inhibited by approximately 60% in both groups treated with the ACE inhibitor, whereas plasma angiotensin converting enzyme activity was reduced only in the Q10 rats. Such results showed that, whereas both hydralazine and quinapril prevented the development of aortic hypertrophy in a pressure-dependent manner, the prevention of the increase in aortic collagen was observed only after ACE inhibition. This latter effect of ACE inhibition was not related to the blood pressure reduction but was associated with the reduction in aortic and not plasma converting enzyme. In a similar protocol using, in addition to quinapril, an angiotensin type I receptor antagonist (CI 996) and the bradykinin antagonist HOE 140, the results indicated that the prevention of aortic collagen accumulation was not due to bradykinin preservation but exclusively to the blockade of angiotensin II type 1 receptors [63]. Interestingly, all these findings are observed under normal or low sodium diet but disappeared in the presence of high sodium diet [64].

Clinical studies

In recent years, noninvasive investigations of large arteries were performed using echo Doppler techniques. In addition, new echo-tracking techniques of high resolution were developed in man to study the inner diameter and the thickness of straight superficial arteries, such as the radial, the brachial and the common carotid arteries [2, 53, 65–70]. Since, in clinical situations, it is not possible to evaluate the whole range of pressure-volume relationships (i.e., from 0 to 200 mmHg), it has been necessary to develop and validate methods for the simultaneous determination of local and systemic dynamic compliance using the determination of pulsatile changes of pressure and diameter [2, 53, 65, 69, 70]. More recently, it has been possible to adequately measure carotid and radial artery wall thickness in humans and to show that both parameters are, on average, increased in untreated hypertensive patients [71, 72]. Under such conditions, the structural abnormalities of large or media-sized arteries may be determined noninvasively in hypertensive subjects, and this may be done before and after drug treatment.

Effect on arterial diameter

In healthy volunteers on an unrestricted sodium diet, increasing doses of the converting enzyme inhibitors perindopril and lisinopril were administered orally [73, 74]. At low doses, ACE inhibition induced preferentially dilatation of arterioles. At higher doses increases in brachial arterial diameter were also obtained. Since plasma converting enzyme activity was blocked even at the lower doses, diameter enlargement of the larger arteries achieved with higher doses of ACE inhibitor were suggested to be rather related to inhibition of tissue converting enzyme.

In patients with sustained essential hypertension, the oral administration of captopril caused a significant acute increase in diameter of the brachial and, to a much lesser extent, the carotid arteries [75]. Like in normotensives, in hypertensives the increase in brachial artery diameter with intravenous perindoprilat was obtained with higher doses than those needed for forearm arteriolar dilatation [2]. With chronic oral administration of the ACE inhibitor, the increase in diameter was maintained during treatment periods of 3–12 months in hypertensive subjects [76, 77]. Since the above findings were obtained in the presence of a significant fall in blood pressure, it seems clear that the dilating effect of ACE inhibition overcame any pressure-related tendency for the arterial diameter to decrease. Depending on the balance between the antihypertensive or the dilating properties, various degrees of diameter change have been obtained with different converting enzyme inhibitors [65, 76, 78–83]. Finally, similar to the results obtained by Caputo et al. from animal experiments [60], clinical studies strongly suggest that in normotensive and hypertensive subjects, converting enzyme inhibition causes a predominant dilatation of peripheral muscular arteries, independent of blood pressure changes [84].

Effect on endothelial function

In humans, the pharmacological effects of converting enzyme inhibition on the arteriolar wall is considered to be mainly due to blockade of the renin angiotensin system. Injections of Ang I and Ang II, in the presence or absence of various converting enzyme inhibitors, into the brachial artery indicate the role of the renin angiotensin system in regulating forearm tone of small arteries

[85]. Other factors may also be involved, like changes in endothelial function with local increases in bradykinin and prostaglandins, and attenuation of sympathetic activity [86–88]. In man, it is possible that each of these factors contributes to large artery dilatation following converting enzyme inhibition. Several of these factors act by influencing endothelium-dependent vasodilation. Indeed, vascular endothelial cells are one of the specific sites of action for bradykinin and converting enzyme [88, 89] and might be involved in producing an increase in brachial artery diameter following converting enzyme inhibition.

In hypertensive subjects, the increase in brachial artery diameter following ACE inhibition is associated with an increase in blood flow velocity [76, 79]. The latter might also contribute to the increase in arterial diameter via the mechanism of high flow dilation which in turn is dependent upon the status of the endothelium. In a long-term study with perindopril in hypertensive subjects [76, 79], the role of flow-dependent dilatation on the brachial artery was evaluated by studying the hemodynamic effects of wrist occlusion at a suprasystolic blood-pressure level. This manoeuver caused a consistent reduction in brachial artery diameter and blood flow velocity during administration of either placebo or ACE inhibition. Although brachial artery diameter decreased with wrist occlusion during active treatment, it remained greater than during placebo administration. These findings support the hypothesis that flow-dependent dilatation and changes in endothelial function accounts in part for the increase in brachial artery diameter, but also suggest that flow-dependent vasodilation is not the only mechanism of action leading to arterial dilatation following ACE inhibition.

Effect on compliance and distensibility

In addition to diameter changes, long-term administration of converting enzyme inhibitors in patients with essential hypertension causes a significant increase in arterial compliance, which was observed at the site of the brachial, radial, femoral and carotid arteries [65, 76, 79, 80, 83]. Several mechanisms may contribute to the increase in compliance. A reduction in blood pressure *per se* lessens the stretch of the arterial wall, thereby favoring an increase in compliance [4]. During converting enzyme inhibition, however, the increase in diameter tends to maintain tangential tension despite the reduction in blood pressure [76, 79]. On the other hand, the direct or indirect effects of converting enzyme inhibition on arterial smooth muscle tone might have favored arterial smooth muscle relaxation with a resulting increase in compliance [84], as has been observed in animal studies [55, 58]. The last possibility is the reversion of arterial structural changes following long-term treatment with converting enzyme inhibitors.

A pioneer study carried out by Kool et al. [65] in subjects with essential hypertension supports the idea that converting enzyme inhibition increases compliance independently of blood pressure level. This study showed that for a similar antihypertensive effect, ACE inhibition improved carotid and femoral compliance whereas hydrochlorothiazide + amiloride had no effect (Fig. 2). A similar finding was observed by Barenbrock et al. [90]. In a randomized double-blind study, the effect of lisinopril and metoprolol on arterial distensibility was studied in patients with hypertension and end-stage renal disease. After a placebo run-in period, the patients were randomly treated with metoprolol (50, 100 or 200 mg) or lisinopril (5, 10 or 20 mg) for ten weeks of therapy. In both groups, a similar antihypertensive effect was observed. Neither ACE inhibition nor beta-blockade influenced the end-diastolic diameter of the common carotid artery after six and ten weeks of treatment. During ACE inhibition, a significant increase in percent change in diameter and distensibility (compared with the metoprolol group) was observed (Fig. 3). An increase in distensibility during ACE inhibition was further confirmed by others [65, 91–95].

In recent years, more direct evidence for the presence of non-pressure related changes in compliance and distensibility resulted from two important findings: the heterogeneity of the arterial response according to the topography of the vessels, and the possible influence of genetic factors. Several studies have shown in hypertensive subjects that, for the same decrease in mean arterial pressure in the whole arterial tree, changes in distensibility differ according to the site of measurements, with major increases in compliance for the brachial artery, the carotid artery and the abdominal aorta whereas no change occurs at

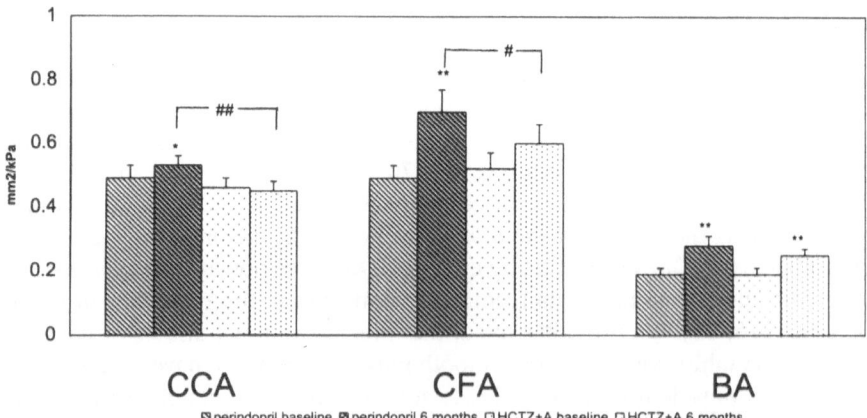

Figure 2. Effect of a six month treatment with perindopril and amiloride/hydrochlorothiazide (A/HCTZ) on arterial compliance of the common carotid artery (CCA), common femoral artery (CFA) and brachial artery (BA). Statistical difference between randomization and six months of treatment: **P < 0.01. Statistical difference in effect at six months between perindopril and amiloride/hydrochlorothiazide: #P < 0.05; ##P < 0.01 [65].

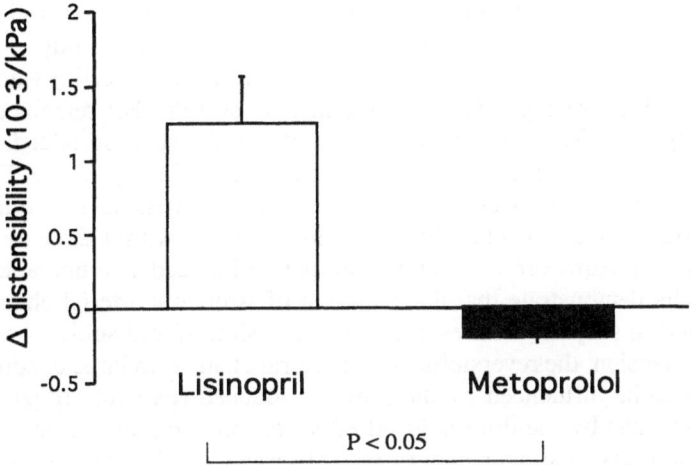

Figure 3. Bar graph shows the change per cent from baseline in distensibility of the common carotid artery after ten weeks of therapy with lisinopril and metoprolol [90] (mean ± SEM).

the site of the radial and the femoral arteries [84, 96–98]. Furthermore, the acute administration of quinapril in hypertensive subjects has shown that, whereas the observed increase of carotid artery distensibility and compliance was clearly pressure-dependent, this was not the case for the total aortic distensibility, demonstrating that, in contrast to the thoracic aorta, the increase in abdominal aorta compliance and distensibility was pressure-independent [96]. Similar findings have been reported using indices of wave reflections as markers of large artery alterations [92, 99]. Finally, it is important to emphasize the role of genetic factors. Benetos et al. [100] have shown the presence of an association between aortic stiffness and AT_1 receptor gene polymorphism. In particular, for the same age and blood pressure, a higher aortic pulse wave velocity was observed in the ac and cc allele subgroups than in the aa subgroup. Furthermore, in hypertensive subjects, the converting enzyme inhibitor perindopril decreased more pulse wave velocity in the (ac + cc) subgroup than in the aa subgroup. This result was found to be independent of blood pressure changes [101]. Because the same results were not found with the calcium entry blocker nitrendipine, it appears that pressure-independent changes in arterial viscoelastic properties may be demonstrated only under converting enzyme inhibition.

Effect on arterial wall thickness

Although a large number of studies exists on changes in vascular structure of small arteries after converting enzyme inhibition or AT_1 blockade [102–105] in hypertension, little is known about the effect on large artery structure in clinical situations [106, 107].

Girerd et al. [108] studied 77 elderly patients with isolated systolic hypertension which were randomized in a double-blind parallel study to receive either perindopril (2–8 mg) or hydrochlorothiazide (HCTZ) + amiloride (HCTZ, 12.5 to 50 mg) over nine months. If systolic BP remained above 160 mmHg after five months, atenolol or chlortalidone were added, respectively. In both groups, there was a similar decrease in blood pressure. The ACE inhibitor significantly decreased radial artery thickness and intima-media cross-sectional area, a result which was not observed within three months of treatment [98]. However, the diuretic compound induced a comparable effect. Such results demonstrate that the reversion of structural arterial changes can be obtained in subjects with essential hypertension. In old subjects with systolic hypertension, the reversibility of structural changes in large conduit arteries seems to be influenced by the pressure-induced (particularly pulse pressure) rather than by the drug-induced effect of treatment on the arterial wall. In these subjects, a similar pattern was observed for the changes in carotid compliance, which increased to the same extent with both drugs. This finding, which differs from that of Kool et al. [65], indicates that different arterial alterations may occur in younger and older hypertensive subjects following drug treatment. Whether this dissimilarity is due to an increased sensitivity to sodium with age or to the well-established decreased reactivity of the renin-angiotensin system with age, or to a combination of both factors remains unknown. In addition, structural alterations of the vessel wall with age leading to a largely irreversible loss of compliance [106] can also limit the effect of an antihypertensive drug on large artery compliance.

Whereas a reduction in wall thickness was observed for the radial artery, no comparable finding was observed for the common carotid artery after converting inhibition by trandolapril for six months [84]. For this musculoelastic artery, there was practically no or little change in carotid artery wall thickness, while diameter was reduced, suggesting arterial remodeling. Similar findings were observed following AT_1 blockade. With this kind of compound, and for the same blood pressure reduction, a significant reduction in radial artery, but not in carotid artery, hypertrophy was achieved [109]. Previous trials have shown that hypercholesterolemic agents markedly decrease carotid artery wall thickness [107], whereas little change is obtained from antihypertensive drugs as calcium entry blockers [110]. Finally, this lack of a significant effect on carotid artery wall thickness contrasts with the rapid reduction in cardiac hypertrophy obtained by converting enzyme inhibitors [76, 84].

Taken together, theses studies clearly indicate that converting enzyme inhibition and even AT_1 receptor blockade have strong effects on the structure and the function of human hypertensive conduit arteries. Apart from the decrease in blood pressure, several of these effects may be due to direct relaxation of arterial smooth muscle and regression of structural changes even if additional endothelial or mechanical factors also seem to be involved.

Prospective views

Hypertension is a cardiovascular risk factor, the mechanisms of which are generally attributed to the reduction in the caliber or number of small arteries or arterioles with a resulting increase in total peripheral resistance and mean blood pressure (MBP). MBP is the product of cardiac output and total peripheral resistance and refers to steady phenomena, considering pressure and flow as constant over time [4]. This definition, based on the description of a steady pressure-flow relationship, does not take into account that blood pressure and flow fluctuate during the cardiac cycle [4]. In clinical practice, pressure is defined in terms of systolic (SBP) and diastolic (DBP) pressure which refer to a pulsatile phenomenon, SBP and DBP representing the extremes of the blood pressure oscillation around a mean value, the MBP. The most modern approach to the blood pressure curve considers arterial pressure as the summation of a steady component, MBP, and a pulsatile component, the pulse pressure (PP). MBP is the pressure for the distribution of steady flow and oxygen to the tissues and organs. The pulsatile component PP is the consequence of the intermittent ventricular ejection from the heart and it is the role of large conduit arteries to minimize the pulsatility.

For many years, only the level of SBP or DBP has been taken into consideration for cardiovascular risk. This means that only the steady, and not the pulsatile, component of blood pressure was considered as the mechanical factor participating in cardiovascular risk. However, it is now widely accepted that pulse pressure is an independent cardiovascular risk factor, mainly for myocardial infarction [48–51], and contributes to the development of clinical [111, 112] and experimental [5] atherosclerosis and to the occurrence of cardiac hypertrophy [113]. Furthermore, increased pulsatile stress is strongly associated with deleterious effects, not only at the site of central conduit arteries, but also at the site of medium-sized arteries and even arterioles [114–116]. On the other hand, in animal experiments, a selective reduction in PP is associated with structural improvement of cerebral and mesenteric arterioles [115]. Thus a specific effect on large arteries may become one of the new important goals of antihypertensive therapy in humans. Both in animals and in humans, there is strong evidence to support this possibility in the cases of ACE inhibition and AT_1 blockade. First, in spontaneously hypertensive rats and in patients with systolic hypertension and end-stage renal disease, converting enzyme inhibition restores the aortic PP amplification normally observed from central to peripheral arteries, causing a more substantial decrease in carotid than in brachial systolic and PP [84, 96, 117, 118]. Secondly, in subjects with essential hypertension, converting enzyme inhibitors may decrease brachial SBP more than β-blocking agents for the same decrease in brachial DBP [119]. Taken together, such results strongly suggest that blockade of the renin-angiotensin system through AT_1 and even AT_2 receptors [120, 121] acts significantly on the large artery system and therefore on the pulsatile component of blood pressure. Further therapeutic trials, particularly in hypertension in the elderly, are needed to investigate this important aspect.

Acknowledgments
This study was performed with the help of INSERM, Association Claude Bernard and GPH-CV. We thank Mrs Anne SAFAR for her skilful technical help.

References

1 Kannel WB, Stokes Jll (1985) Hypertension as a cardiovascular risk factor. *In*: Bulpitt CJ (ed.): *Handbook of Hypertension Epidemiology of Hypertension*. Elsevier Science, Amsterdam, 15–34
2 Safar ME, London GM (1994) The arterial system in human hypertension. *In*: JD Swales (ed:). *Textbook of hypertension*. Blackwell Scientific, London, 85–102
3 Gibbons GH, Dzau VJ (1994) The emerging concept of vascular remodelling. *N Engl J Med* 330: 1431–1438
4 Nichols WW, O'Rourke MF (1998) McDonald's blood flow in arteries. Theoretical, experimental and clinical principles. E Arnold, Fourth edition. London, Sydney, Auckland, 54–113, 201–222, 284–292: 347–401
5 Glagov S, Weidenberg E, Zarins CK, Stankunavicius R, Kolettis GJ (1987) Compensatory enlargement of human atherosclerotic coronary arteries. *N Engl J Med* 316: 1371–1375
6 Girerd X, London G, Boutouyrie P, Mourad J-J, Safar M, Laurent S (1996) Remodelling of radial artery in response to a chronic increase in shear stress. *Hypertension* 27 (part 2): 799–803
7 Davies PF (1995) Flow-mediated endothelial mechanotransduction. *Physiol Rev* 75: 519–560
8 Traub O, Berk BC (1998) Laminar shear stress: mechanisms by which endothelial cells transduce an atheroprotective force. *Arterioscler Thromb Vasc Biol* 18: 677–685
9 Moncada S, Palmer RMJ, Higgs EA (1991) Nitric oxide: physiology, pathophysiology and pharmacology. *Pharmacol Rev* 43: 109–142
10 Dzau VJ (1993) The role of mechanical and humoral factors in growth regulation of vascular smooth muscle and cardiac myocytes. *Curr Opin Nephrol Hypertens* 2: 27–32
11 Birukov KG, Bardy N, Lehoux S, Merval R, Shirinsky VP, Tedgui A (1998) Intraluminal pressure is essential for the maintenance of smooth muscle calmodesmon and filamin content in aortic organ culture. *Arterioscler Thromb Vasc Biol* 18: 922–927
12 Glagov S, Vito R, Giddens DP, Zarins Ch K (1992) Micro-architecture and composition of artery walls: relationship to location, diameter and the distribution of mechanical stress. *J Hypertension* 10 (suppl 6),: S101–S104
13 Schwartz SM, Heimark RL, Majesty MW (1990) Developmental mechanisms underlying pathology of arteries. *Physiol Rev* 70: 1177–1198
14 Mulvany MJ (1987) The structure of the resistance vasculature in essential hypertension. *J Hypertension* 5: 129–136
15 Mourad J-J, Girerd X, Boutouyrie P, Safar M, Laurent S (1998) Opposite effects of remodelling and hypertrophy on arterial compliance in hypertension. *Hypertension* 31 (part 2): 529–533
16 Partovian C, Benetos A, Pommies JP, Safar ME (1998) Effects of a chronic high-salt diet on large artery structure: role of endogenous bradykinin. *Amer J Physiol* 274: (*Heart Circ Physiol* 43): H1423–H1428
17 Fischer GM, Swain ML (1978) *In vivo* effects of sex hormones on aortic elastin and collagen dynamics in castrated and intact male rats. *Endocrinology* 102: 92–97
18 Unger T, Chung O, Csikos T, Culman J, Gallinat S, Gohlke P, Meffert S, Stoll M, Stroth U et al (1996) Angiotensin receptors. *J Hypertension* 14 (suppl 5): S95–S103
19 Penit J, Faure M, Alfert JS (1983) Vasopressin and angiotensin II receptors in rat aortic smooth muscle cells in culture. *Amer J Physiol* 244: E72–E82
20 Folkow B, Grimby G, Thulesius O (1958) Adaptative structural changes of the vascular wall in hypertension and their relation to the control of the peripheral resistance. *Acta Physiol Scand* 44: 255–272

21 Dzau VJ, Safar ME (1977) Large arteries in hypertension: role of the renin-angiotensin system. *Circulation* 77: 947–953

22 Lever AF (1986) Slow pressor mechanisms in hypertension: a role for hypertrophy of resistance vessels? *J Hypertension* 4: 515–524

23 Bunkenburg B, Van Amelsvoort T, Rogg H, Wood JM (1992) Receptor-mediated effects of angiotensin II on growth of vascular smooth muscle cells from spontaneously hypertensive rats. *Hypertension* 20: 746–754

24 Arnal JF, Battle T, Rasetti C, Challah M, Costerousse O, Vicaut E, Michel JG, Alhenc-Gelas F (1994) ACE in three tunicae of rat aorta: expression in smooth muscle and effect of renovascular hypertension. *Amer J Physiol* 267: H1777–H1784

25 Gohlke P, Bunning P, Unger T (1992) Distribution and metabolism of angiotensin I and II in the blood vessel wall. *Hypertension* 20: 151–157

26 Geisterfer AAT, Peach MJ, Owens GK (1988) Angiotensin II induces hypertrophy, not hyperplasia, of cultured rat aortic smooth muscle cells. *Circ Res* 62: 749–756

27 Morichita R, Gibbons GH, Ellison KE, Lee W, Zhang L, Yu H, Kaneda Y, Ogihara T, Dzau VJ (1994) Evidence for direct local effect of angiotensin In vascular hypertrophy. *In vivo* gene transfer of angiotensin converting enzyme. *J Clin Invest* 94: 978–984

28 Kato H, Suzuki H, Tajima S, Ogata Y, Tominaga T, Sato A, Saruta T (1991) Angiotensin II stimulates collagen synthesis in cultured vascular smooth muscle cells. *J Hypertension* 9: 17–22

29 Griffin SA, Brown WCB, Macpherson F, Macgrath JC, Wilson VG, Korsgaard N, Mulvany MJ, Lever AF (1991) Angiotensin II causes vascular hypertrophy in part by a non pressor mechanism. *Hypertension* 17: 626–635

30 Simon G, Altman S (1992) Subpressor angiotensin II is a bifunctional growth factor of vascular muscle in rats. *J Hypertension* 10: 1165–1171

31 Guyton JR, Hartley CJ (1985) Flow restriction of one carotid artery in juvenile rats exhibits growth of arterial diameter. *Amer J Physiol* 248: H540–H546

32 Langille BL, O'Donnell F (1986) Reductions in arterial diameters produced by chronic decrease in blood flow are endothelium-dependent. *Science* 231: 405–407

33 Tohda K, Masuda H, Kawamura K, Shozawa T (1992) Difference in dilatation between endothelium-preserved and -desquamated segments in the flow-loaded rat common carotid artery. *Arterioscler Thromb* 12: 519–528

34 Bassiouny HS, Zarins CK, Kadowaki MH, Glagov S (1994) Hemodynamic stress and experimental aortoiliac atherosclerosis. *J Vasc Surg* 19: 426–434

35 Cunha R, Dabire H, Bezie I, Weiss AM, Chaouche-Teyara K, Laurent S, Safar M, Lacolley P (1997) Mechanical stress of the carotid artery at the early phase of spontaneous hypertension in rats. *Hypertension* 29: 992–998

36 Levy BI, Benessiano J, Poitevin P, Safar ME (1990) Endothelium-dependent mechanical properties of carotid artery in WKY and SHR: role of angiotensin converting enzyme inhibition. *Circ Res* 66: 321–328

37 Levy BI, El Fertak L, Pieddeloup C, Barouki F, Safar ME (1993) Role of endothelium in the mechanical response of the carotid arterial wall to calcium blockade in spontaneous hypertensive and Wiskar-Kyoto rats. *J Hypertension* 11: 57–63

38 Krooker EJ, Wood EH (1955) Comparison of simultaneously recorded central and peripheral arterial pressure pulses during rest, exercise and tilded position in man. *Circ Res* 3: 623–632

39 Pohl U, Holtz J, Busse R, Bassenge E (1986) Crucial role of endothelium in the vasodilator response to the increased flow *in vivo*. *Hypertension* 8: 37–44

40 Laurent S, Girerd X, Mourad JJ, Lacolley P, Beck L, Boutouyrie P, Mignot JP, Safar M (1994) Elastic modulus of the radial artery wall material is not increased in patients with essential hypertension. *Arterioscler Thromb* 14: 1223–1233

41 London GM, Guerin AP, Marchais SJ, Pannier B, Safar ME, Day M, Metivier F (1996) Cardiac and arterial interactions in end-stage renal disease. *Kidney Int* 50: 600–608

42 Hoeks APG, Brands PJ, Smeets Gam, Reneman RS (1990) Assessment of the distensibility of superficial arteries *Ultrasound. Med Biol* 16: 121–128

43 Kelly R, Hayward C, Ganis J, Daley J, Avolio A, O'Rourke MF (1989) Non-invasive registration of the arterial pressure pulse waveform using high-fidelity applanation tonometry. *J Vasc Med* 1: 142–149

44 Chen CH, Nevo E, Fetics B, Pak PH, Yin FCP, Maughan L, Kass DE (1997) Estimation of central aortic pressure waveform by mathematical transformation of radial tonometry pressure. Validation

of generalized transfer function. *Circulation* 95: 1827–1836

45 Avolio AO, Chen SG, Wang RP, Zhang CI, Li MF, O'Rourke MF (1983) Effect of aging on changing arterial compliance and left ventricular load in northern chinese urban community. *Circulation* 68: 50–58

46 Bramwell JV, Hill AV (1922) Velocity of transmission of the pulse wave and elasticity of arteries. *Lancet* 1: 891–892

47 London GM, Yaginuma T (1993) Wave reflections: clinical, therapeutic aspects. *In*: ME Safar, MF O'Rourke (ed.): *The arterial system in hypertension*. Kluwer Academic, Dordrecht, Boston, London, 221–237

48 Darné B, Girerd X, Safar M, Cambien F, Guize L (1989) Pulsatile *versus* steady component of blood pressure: A cross-sectional analysis and a prospective analysis on cardiovascular mortality. *Hypertension* 13: 392–400

49 Madhavan S, Ooi WL, Cohen H, Alderman MH (1994) Relation of pulse pressure and blood pressure reduction to the incidence of myocardial infarction. *Hypertension* 23: 395–401

50 Benetos A, Safar M, Rudnichi A, Smulyan H, Richard JL, Ducimetiere P, Guize L (1997) Pulse pressure: a predictor of long-term cardiovascular mortality in a french male population. *Hypertension* 30: 1410–1415

51 Mitchell GF, Moye LM, Braunwald E, Rouleau J-L, Bernstein V, Geltman EM, Flaker GC, Pfeffer MA, the Saveinvestigators (1997) Sphygmomanometrically determined pulse pressure is a powerful independent predictor of recurrent events after myocardial infarction in patients with impaired left ventricular function. *Circulation* 96: 4254–4260

52 Cox RH (1981) Basis for the altered arterial wall mechanics in the spontaneously hypertensive rat. *Hypertension* 3: 485–495

53 Hayoz D, Rutschmann B, Perret F, Niederberger M, Tardy Y, Mooser V, Nussberger J, Waeber B, Brunner H (1992) Conduit artery compliance and distensibility are not necessarily reduced in hypertension. *Hypertension* 20: 1–6

54 Armentano R, Megnien JL, Simon A, Bellenfant F, Barra J, Levenson J (1995) Effects of hypertension on viscoelasticity of carotid and femoral arteries in humans. *Hypertension* 26: 48–54

55 Levy BI, Michel JL, Salzmann JL, Azizi M, Poitevin F, Safar ME, Camilleri JP (1988) Effects of chronic inhibition of converting enzyme on mechanical and structural properties of arteries in rat renovascular hypertension. *Circ Res*, 63: 227–229

56 Van Gorp AW, Van Ingen Schenau DS, Hoeks AP, Struijker Boudier HA (1995) Aortic wall properties in normotensive and hypertensive rats of various ages *in vivo. Hypertension* 26 (2): 363–368

57 Liu Z, Ting C-T, Zhu S, Yin Fcp (1989) Aortic compliance in human hypertension. *Hypertension* 140: 129–136

58 Levy BI, Michel JL, Salzmann JL, Poitevin F, Devissaguet M, Scalbert E, Safar ME (1993) Long-term effects of angiotensin-converting enzyme inhibition on the arterial wall of adult spontaneously hypertensive rats. *Amer J Cardiol* 71: E8–E16

59 Benetos A, Pannier B, Brahimi M, Safar ME, Levy BI (1993) Dose-related changes in the mechanical properties of the carotid artery in WKY rats and SHR following relaxation of arterial smooth muscle. *J Vasc Res* 30: 23–29

60 Caputo L, Tedgui A, Levy BI (1995) Control of carotid vasomotor tone by local renin-angiotensin system in normotensive and spontaneously hypertensive rats: role of endothelium and flow. *Circ Res* 77: 303–309

61 Benetos A, Elfertak L, Safar M, Levy B (1991) Effects of bradykinin on carotid artery compliance: the role of the endothelium. *J Hypertension* 9 (suppl 6): S204–S205

62 Albaladejo P, Bouaziz H, Duriez M, Gohlke P, Levy B, Safar M, Benetos A (1994) Angiotensin converting enzyme inhibition prevents the increase in aortic collagen in rats. *Hypertension* 23: 74–82

63 Benetos A, Levy BI, Lacolley P, Taillard F, Duriez M, Safar ME (1997) Role of angiotensin II and bradykinin on aortic collagen following converting-enzyme inhibition in spontaneously hypertensive rats. *Arterioscler Thromb Vasc Biol* 17: 3196–3201

64 Labat C, Lacolley P, Koffi I, Ledulal K, Safar ME, Benetos A (1999) AT1 blockade of angiotensine II and sodium diet: effect on carotid artery structure and function in SHRs. *J Hypertension* 17 (suppl 3): S131

65 Kool MJ, Lusterman FA, Breed JG, Struyker Boudier HA, Hoeks AP, Reneman RS, Van Bortel LM (1995) The influence of perindopril and the diuretic combination amiloride + hydrochlorothiazide on the vessel wall properties of large arteries in hypertensive patients. *J Hypertension* 13:

839–848

66 Chau NP, Simon A, Vilar J, Cabrera-Fisher E, Pithois-Merli I, Levenson J (1992) Active and passive effects of antihypertensive drugs on large artery diameter and elasticity in human essential hypertension. *J Cardiovasc Pharmacol* 19: 78–85

67 Barra JG, Armentano RL, Levenson J, Cabrera-Fisher EI, Pichel RH, Simon A (1993) Assessment of smooth muscle contribution to descending thoracic aorta elastic mechanics in conscious dogs. *Circ Res* 73: 1040–1050

68 Heintz B, Walkenhorst F, Gillessen T, Dorr R, Krebs W, Vom Dahl J, Hanrath P (1994) *In vivo* characterization of segmental elastic properties of the aortic tree by intravascular ultrasound. *Cardiol Elderl* 2: 127–131

69 Laurent S, Caviezel B, Beck L, Girerd X, Billaud E, Boutouyrie P, Hoeks A, Safar M (1994) Carotid artery distensibility and distending pressure in hypertensive humans. *Hypertension* 23 (part II): 878–883

70 Kool MJF, Van Merode T, Reneman RS, Hoeks APG, Struijker Boudier Haj, Van Bortel Lmab (1994) Evaluation of reproducibility of a vessel wall movement detector system for assessment of large properties. *Cardiovasc Res* 28: 610–614

71 Roman MJ, Saba PS, Pini R, Spitzer M, Pickering TG, Rosen S, Alderman MH, Devereux RB (1992) Parallel cardiac and vascular adaptation in hypertension. *Circulation* 86: 1909–1918

72 Girerd X, Mourad J-J, Copie X, Moulin C, Acar C, Safar M, Laurent S (1994) Non invasive detection of an increased vascular mass in untreated hypertensive patients. *Amer J Hypertens* 7: 1076–1084

73 Richer C, Thuilliez C, Giudicelli JP (1987) Perindopril, converting enzyme blockade, and peripheral arterial hemodynamics in the healthy volunteer. *J Cardiovasc Pharmacol* 9: 94–102

74 Perret F, Mooser V, Hayoz D, Tardy Y, Meister JJ, Etienne JD, Farine PA, Marazzi A, Burnier M, Nussberger J et al (1991) Evaluation of arterial compliance-pressure curves; effect of antihypertensive drugs. *Hypertension* 18 (suppl II): II77–II83

75 Bouthier JD, Safar ME, Benetos A, Simon A, Levenson JA, Hugue Ch (1986) Hemodynamic effects of vasodilating drugs on the common carotid and brachial circulations of patients with essential hypertension. *Brit J Clin Pharmacol* 21: 136–142

76 Asmar RG, Pannier B, Santoni JP, Laurent ST, London GM, Levy BI, Safar ME (1988) Reversion of cardiac hypertrophy and reduced arterial compliance after converting enzyme inhibition in essential hypertension. *Circulation* 78: 941–950

77 Asmar RG, Journo HK, Lacolley PJ, Santoni JP, Billaud E, Safar ME (1988) One year treatment with perindopril: effect on cardiac mass and arterial compliance in essential hypertension. *J Hypertension* 6 (suppl 3): 33–39

78 Asmar R, Benetos A, Brahimi M, Chaouche K, Safar M (1992) Arterial and antihypertensive effects of nitrendipine: a double-blind comparison *versus* placebo. *J Cardiovasc Pharmacol* 20: 858–863

79 Asmar RG, Journo HJ, Lacolley PJ, Santoni JP, Billaud B, Levy BI, Safar ME (1988) Treatment for one year with perindopril: effects on cardiac mass and arterial compliance in essential hypertension. *J Hypertension* 6 (suppl 3): S33–S39

80 De Luca N, Savonitto S, Riciardelli B, Marchegiano R, Lamenza F, Lembo G, Trimarco B (1993) Effects of the single and repeated administration of benazepril on systemic and forearm circulation and cardiac function in hypertensive patients. *Cardiovasc Drug Therapy* 7: 211–216

81 Giannattasio C, Faila M, Stella ML, Mangoni A, Turrini D, Carugo S, Pozzi M, Grassi G, Mancia G (1995) Angiotensin-converting enzyme inhibition and radial artery compliance in patients with congestive heart failure. *Hypertension* 26: 491–496

82 Bellissant E, Thuillez C, Richer C, Pussard E, Giudicelli JF (1994) Noninvasive assessment of regional arteriolar and arterial dilating properties of lisonopril in healthy volunteers. *J Cardiovasc Pharmacol* 24: 500–506

83 De Luca N, Rosiello G, Lamenza F, Riciardelli B, Marchegiano R, Volpe M, Marelli C, Trimarco B (1992) Reversal of cardiac and large artery structural abnormalities induced by long-term antihypertensive treatment with trandolapril. *Amer J Cardiol* 70: 52D–59D

84 Topouchian J, Asmar R, Sayeg F, Rudnicki A, Benetos A, Bacri AM, Safar ME (1999) Changes in arterial structure and function under trandolapril-verapamil combination in hypertension. *Stroke* 30: 1056–1064

85 Webb DJ, Benjamin N, Cockcroft JR, Collier JG (1989) Augmentation of sympathetic venoconstriction by angiotensin II in human dorsal hand veins. *Amer J Hypertens* 2: 721–723

86 Qiu YY, Henrion D, Levy BI (1994) Endogenous angiotensin II enhances phenylephrine-induced tone in hypertensive rats. *Hypertension* 24: 317–321

87 Stefas L, Levy BI (1991) Effects of saralasin on arterial compliance in normotensive and hypertensive rats; role of endothelium. *Hypertension* 18 (suppl II): 79–83

88 Mombouli JV, Vanhoutte PM (1992) Heterogeneity of endothelium-dependent vasodilator effects of angiotensin-converting enzyme inhibitors: role of bradykinin generation during ACE inhibition. *J Cardiovasc Pharmacol* (suppl 9): S79–S83

89 Mombouli JV, Iliano S, Nagao T, Scott-Burden T, Vanhoutte PM (1992) Potentiation of endothelium-dependent, relaxations to bradykinin by angiotensin 1 converting enzyme inhibitors in canine coronary artery involves both endothelium derived relaxing and hyperpolarizing factors. *Circ Res* 71: 137–144

90 Barenbrock M, Spieker C, Hoeks APG, Ziedekw, Rahn KH (1994) Effect of lisinopril and metoprolol on arterial distensibility. *Hypertension* 24 (suppl I): I-161–I-163

91 Shimamoto H, Shimamoto Y (1995) Lisinopril improves aortic compliance and renal flow. Comparison with nifedipine. *Hypertension* 25: 327–334

92 Chen CH, Ting CT, Lin SJ, Hsu FCP, Siu CO, Chou P, Wang SP, Chang MS (1995) Different effects of fosinopril and atenolol on wave reflections in hypertension. *Hypertension* 25: 1034–1041

93 Savolainen A, Keto P, Poutanen VP, Hekali P, Standertskjold-Nordenstam CG, Rames A, Kupari M (1996) Effects of angiotensin-converting enzyme inhibition *versus* beta-adrenergic blockade on aortic stiffness in essential hypertension. *J Cardiovasc Pharmacol* 27: 99–104

94 Schartl M, Bocksch WG, Dreysse S, Beckmann S, Franke O, Uunten U (1994) Remodeling of myocardium and arteries by chronic angiotensin converting enzyme inhibition in hypertensive patients. *J Hypertension* 12 (suppl 4): S37–S42

95 DECesaris R, Ranieri G, Filitti V, Andirani A, Bonfantino MV (1993) Forearm arterial distensibility in patients with hypertension: comparative effects of long-term ACE inhibition and beta-blocking agents. Pharmacodynamics and drug action. *Clin Pharmacol Ther* 53: 360–367

96 Topouchian J, Brisac AM, Pannier B, Vicaut E, Safar M, Asmar R (1998) Assessment of the acute arterial effects of converting enzyme inhibition in essential hypertension: a double-blind, comparative and cross-over study. *J Hum Hypertens* 12: 181–187

97 Benetos A, Lafleche A, Asmar R, Gautier S, Safar A, Safar ME (1996) Arterial stiffness, hydrochlorothiazide and converting enzyme inhibition in essential hypertension. *J Hum Hypertens* 10: 77–82

98 Lafleche A, Gautier S, Topouchian J, Wilmet CS, Girerd X, Safar ME, Benetos A (1998) Differential responses of the heart and vasculature to chronic blood pressure reduction in essential hypertension. *Clin Pharmacol* 64: 96–105

99 London G, Pannier B, Vicaut E, Guerin AP, Marchais SJ, Safar ME, Cuche JL (1996) Antihypertensive effects and arterial hemodynamic alterations during ACE inhibition. *J Hypertension* 14: 1139–1146

100 Benetos A, Gauthier S, Ricard S, Topouchian J, Asmar R, Poirier O, Larosa E, Guize L, Safar M, Soubrier F et al (1996) Influence of angiotensin-converting enzyme and angiotensin II type I receptor gene polymorphisms on aortic stiffness in normotensive and hypertensive patients. *Circulation* 94: 698–703

101 Benetos A, Cambien F, Gautier S, Ricard S, Safar ME, Laurent S, Lacolley P, Poirier O, Topouchian J, Asmar R (1996) Influence of the angiotensin type 1 receptor gene polymorphism on the effects of perindopril and nitrendipine on arterial stiffness in hypertensive individuals. *Hypertension* 28: 1081–1084

102 Morton JJ, Beattie EC, Macpherson F (1992) Angiotensin II receptor antagonist losartan has persistent effect on blood pressure in the young spontaneously hypertensive rat: lack of relaxation to vascular structure. *J Vasc Res* 29: 264–269

103 Shaw LM, Geaorge PR, Oldham AA, Heagerty AM (1995) A comparison of the effect of angiotensin converting enzyme inhibition and angiotensin II receptor antagonism on structural changes associated with hypertension in rat small arteries. *J Hypertension* 13: 1135–1144

104 Li J-S, Sharifi AM, Schiffrin EL (1997) Effect of AT1 angiotensin-receptor blockade on structure and function of small arteries in SHR. *J Cardiovasc Pharmacol* 30: 75–83

105 Rizzoni D, Porteri E, Bettoni G, Piccoli A, Castellano M, Muiesan ML, Pasini G, Guelfi D, Rosei EA (1998) Effects of candesartan cilexetil and enalapril on structural alterations and endothelial function in small resistance arteries of spontaneously hypertensive rats. *J Cardiovasc Pharmacol*

32: 798–806

106 Van Bortel LM, Hoeks APG, Kool MJF, Struijker-Boudier HAJ (1992) Introduction to large artery properties as a target for risk reduction by antihypertensive therapy. *J Hypertension* 10 (suppl 6): 123–126

107 Safar ME, Girerd X, Laurent S (1996) Structural changes of large conduit arteries in hypertension. *J Hypertension* 14: 545–555

108 Girerd X, Giannattasio C, Moulin C, Safar M, Mancia G, Laurent S (1998) Regression of radial artery wall hypertrophy and improvement of carotid artery compliance after long-term antihypertensive treatment in elderly patients *J Amer Coll Cardiol*, 31: 1064–1073

109 Benetos A, Gautier S, Lafleche A, Topouchian J, Guyen TT, Frangin G, Girerd X, Sissmann J, Safar ME (2000) AT1 blockade of angiotensin II: effect on carotid and radial arterial structure and function in hypertensive humans. *J Vasc Res* 37: 8–15

110 Borhani NO, Mercuri M, Borhani PA, Buckalew VM, Canossa-Terris M, Carr AA, Kappagoda T, Rocco MV, Schnaper HW, Sowers JR et al (1996) Final outcome results of the Multicenter Isradipine Diuretic Atherosclerosis Study (MIDAS). A randomized controlled trial. *J Amer Med Assn* 276: 785–791

111 Safar ME, Toto-Moukouo JJ, Asmar RA, Laurent ST (1987) Increased pulse pressure in patients with arteriosclerosis obliterans of the lower limb. *Arteriosclerosis* 7: 232–237

112 Asmar RG, Girerd XJ, Brahimi M, Safavian A, Safar ME (1992) Ambulatory blood pressure measurement, smoking and abnormalities of glucose and lipid metabolism in essential hypertension. *J Hypertension* 10: 181–187

113 Pannier B, Brunel P, ELAroussy W, Lacolley P, Safar ME (1989) Pulse pressure and echocardiographic findings in essential hypertension. *J Hypertension* 7: 127–129

114 Baumbach GL, Siems JE, Heistad DD (1991) Effects of local reduction in pressure on distensibility and composition of cerebral arterioles. *Circ Res* 68: 339–351

115 Christensen KL (1991) Reducing pulse pressure in hypertension may normalize small artery structure. *Hypertension* 18: 722–727

116 Baumbach GL (1996) Effects of increased pulse pressure on cerebral arterioles. *Hypertension* 27: 159–167

117 London GM, Pannier B, Guerin AP, Marchais SJ, Safar ME, Cuche JJ (1994) Cardiac hypertrophy, aortic compliance, peripheral resistance, and wave reflection in end-stage renal disease. Comparative effects of ACE inhibition and calcium channel blockade. *Circulation* 90: 2786–2796

118 Tsoucaris D, Benetos A, Legrand M, London G, Safar M (1995) Proximal and distal pulse pressure after acute antihypertensive vasodilating drugs in Wistar-Kyoto and spontaneously hypertensive rats. *J Hypertension* 13: 243–249

119 Pannier B, Garabedian VG, Madonna O, Fouchard M, Darné B, Safar ME (1991) Lisinopril *versus* atenolol: decrease in systolic *versus* diastolic blood pressure with converting enzyme inhibition. *Cardiovasc Drug Therapy* 5: 775–782

120 Sabri A, Levy BI, Poitevin P, Caputo L, Faggin E, Marotte F, Rappaport L, Samuel JL (1997) Differential roles of AT_1 and AT_2 receptor subtypes in vascular trophic and phenotypic changes in response to stimulation with angiotensin II. *Arterioscler Thromb Vasc Biol* 17: 257–264

121 Levy BI, Benessiano J, Henrion D, Caputo L, Heymes C, Duriez M, Poitevin P, and Samuel JL (1996) Chronic blockade of AT_2 subtype receptors prevents the effect of angiotensin II on the rat vascular structure. *J Clin Invest* 98: 418–425

ACE Inhibitors
ed. by P. D'Orléans-Juste and G.E. Plante
© 2001 Birkhäuser Verlag/Switzerland

The contribution of angiotensin-converting enzyme (ACE) to the metabolism of kinins (bradykinin and des-Arg^9-bradykinin) and effect of ACE inhibitors on their *in vitro* and *in vivo* metabolism

Albert Adam[1], Charles Blais, Jr.[1] and François Marceau[2]

[1] *Faculté de pharmacie, Université de Montréal, Montréal, QC, H3C 3J7, Canada*
[2] *Centre Hospitalier Universitaire de Québec, Centre de recherche du Pavillon L'Hôtel-Dieu de Québec, Québec, QC, G1R 2J6, Canada*

Introduction: the kallikrein-kinin system

Similar to the renin-angiotensin system, the kallikrein-kinin system (KKS) is a cascade system of activators (kallikreins) which hydrolyse substrates (kininogens) to release vasoactive peptides (kinins). The nature of the various constituents and their properties have been extensively reviewed recently [1]. Low and high molecular weight kininogens (LK and HK, respectively) are multidomained and multifunctional glycoproteins which exert various regulatory functions at sites of local inflammation. They release kinins which are powerful proinflammatory peptides and also inhibit, at least *in vitro*, lysosomal thiol proteases released during tissue injury. Through its light chain, HK is a cofactor in the activation of Hageman factor by contact with a negatively charged surface (e.g., damaged myocardium) which leads to the formation of a clot.

Kinins are released from kininogens by specific plasma and tissue kallikreins and by non-specific serine proteases. The major native kinins released are bradykinin (BK) and Lys-BK (kallidin). Various peptidases are capable of metabolizing kinins, among which angiotensin I-converting enzyme (ACE, kininase II, dipeptidyl carboxypeptidase, peptidyldipeptide hydrolase, EC 3.4.15.1) plays an important role [2] (Fig. 1). All these peptidases inactivate the pharmacological activity of BK, except kininase I, a generic name for carboxypeptidases, which transforms BK and Lys-BK to their des-Arg^9-metabolites.

Kinins are proinflammatory peptides. They cause vasodilation and vasopermeability and also stimulate nociceptive fibers. They exert their pharmacological activity by activating two types of G protein–coupled receptors: the B$_1$ subtype, selectively stimulated by the des-Arg^9-metabolites, and B$_2$ receptors,

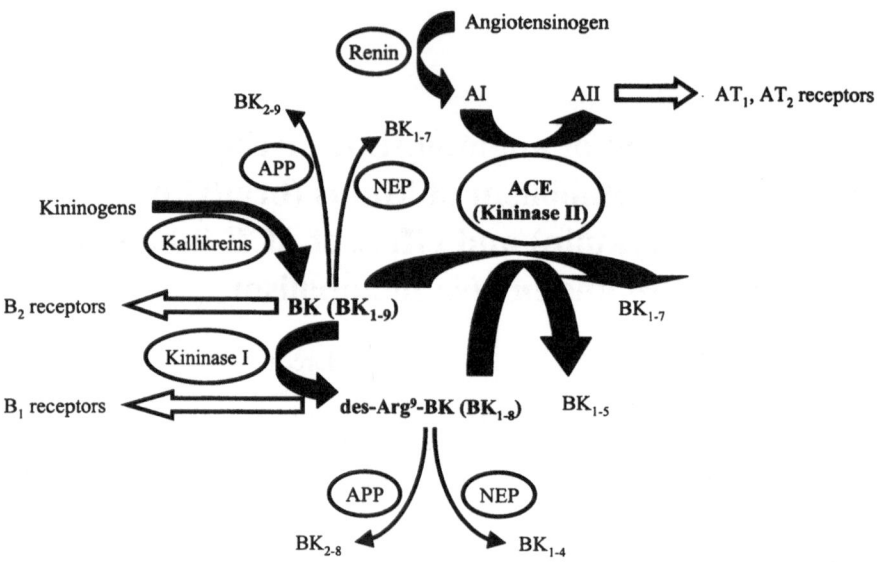

Figure 1. Some of the metabolic pathways postulated to be important for the physiology of vasoactive peptides (see text). Abbreviations: ACE: angiotensin-converting enzyme; AI: angiotensin I; AII: angiotensin II; APP: aminopeptidase P; BK: bradykinin; NEP: neutral endopeptidase 24.11; White arrows: receptor stimulation; Black arrows: enzymatic cleavage. The metabolites mentioned in the figure are the first to be generated by enzyme activity.

for which the native kinins BK and Lys-BK are the optimal agonists [3]. In addition to differences in the structure of their specific agonists, B_1 and B_2 receptors differ in the regulation of their expression. B_2 receptors are preformed and widely distributed in normal tissues while B_1 receptor gene expression is profoundly regulated, to the point that it is a completely inducible gene under the control of the cytokine network and the mitogen-activated protein kinases controlled by cell injury [4]. Thus, B_1 receptor expression may be limited to pathological conditions. B_1 and B_2 receptors have been cloned and exhibit a modest degree of homology (36% identity at the amino acid sequence level). The stimulation of either B_1 or B_2 receptors at the endothelial level leads to the activation of phospholipase C and A_2, and to the release of prostaglandins (PGs), typically PGI_2 and PGE_2, and of nitric oxide (NO), via the activation of key calcium-sentitive enzymes (cytosolic phospholipase A_2, endothelial NO synthase). NO in turn is responsible for the generation of cGMP in the neighbouring cells, and the anti-proliferative properties of BK are attributed to the latter signaling system [5, 6]. Whether normal or pathological autoregulation of the circulation recruits the vasodilator effect of kinins in peripheral tissues is a crucial issue for which there is little published evidence, especially in humans. However, much of the literature on the KKS relationship to ACE inhibitors (ACEi) is based on the assumption that the beneficial vasodilator effect of kinins can be dissociated from their inflammatory effects (e.g., increased local vascular permeability and lymphatic flow, reflex tachycardia produced by BK-stimulated visceral afferent neurons [7]).

Although liver and kidney are the main sites of synthesis of the KKS, constituents of this system are also seen in blood vessels [8], heart [9], endothelial cells [10] and cardiomyocytes [11]. For these reasons, and also due to their high susceptibility to hydrolysis (see below), kinins are now considered as autocrine and paracrine factors rather than hormones.

In this chapter, we will critically review recent findings on the analytical biochemistry and pharmacology of the kinins (BK and des-Arg^9-BK) in relation to the therapeutic and side effects of ACEi.

Kinins: natural substrates for purified ACE

As early as in 1967, Ferreira and Vane [12] reported that the biological activity of BK disappeared during passage through the pulmonary circulation. Ferreira [13] demonstrated that a peptide mixture isolated from the venom of *Bothrops jararaca* inhibits the degradation of BK and potentiates its action on the smooth muscle. Bakhle [14] originally demonstrated that the same mixture of peptides inhibited the formation of angiotensin I (AI) by a canine pulmonary preparation. These observations led Ng and Vane [15] to suggest that the same pulmonary enzyme might catalyze AI conversion and BK inactivation (Fig. 1).

Substrate specificity

In 1980, Cushman and Ondetti [16] showed that BK is a substrate for ACE. This enzyme sequentially cleaves two carboxy-terminal dipeptides from BK (Phe–Arg and Ser–Pro successively), transforming the B$_2$ agonist into the inactive final product BK$_{1-5}$. In addition to BK, ACE can also metabolize BK$_{1-7}$ and amino-extended homologues of BK (Lys–BK and Met–Lys–BK), although the rates of hydrolysis are much lower than that of BK [17]. Not only the B$_2$, but also B$_1$ receptor agonists are natural substrates for ACE. Specifically, ACE metabolizes des-Arg^9-BK by releasing the carboxy-terminal tripeptide Ser–Pro–Phe, thus yielding the same BK$_{1-5}$ end product as BK [18].

The influence of various physicochemical parameters on the catalytic activity of ACE has been studied. As for AI, hydrolysis of BK is activated by Cl$^-$ anions. However, in contrast to the reaction involving AI, the optimal concentration of Cl$^-$ is much lower for BK (20 mM, instead of 200 mM for AI). Moreover, in the absence of chloride, about 45% of the maximal kininase activity of ACE is retained [19].

Kinetic parameters

When compared with the kinetic parameters of the reaction that produces angiotensin II (AII) from AI, it appears that ACE has a higher affinity for BK and des-Arg^9-BK [18, 20–25]. Different values of K_m and k_{cat}/K_m have been reported in the literature. Using a recombinant human ACE, Jaspard et al. [26, 27] have calculated a K_m and a k_{cat}/K_m, respectively, equal to 0.18 μM and 61×10^{-6} M^{-1} s^{-1} for BK against 16 μM and 2.2×10^{-6} M^{-1} s^{-1} for AI. These findings have incited some authors to consider ACE primarily as a kininase rather than an angiotensinase [21].

The kininase activity of the two catalytic sites of ACE

The kininase activity of both amino- and carboxy-catalytic domains of ACE has been carefully characterized by Jaspard et al. [27]. Both active sites metabolize BK, however, with different kinetic parameters. For instance, the amino-domain accounts for almost 25% of the total kininase activity of ACE and the carboxy-domain for almost 75%. The two sites exhibit a different sensitivity to Cl$^-$. The concentration of Cl$^-$ anions also influences the nature of the final metabolites (BK$_{1-7}$ or BK$_{1-5}$) and their relative concentrations.

Role of ACE in the metabolism of kinins in various biological milieus

The multiple peptidases capable of metabolizing kinins have been recently extensively reviewed by Erdös and Skidgel [2]. Although various purified peptidases metabolize kinins, the K_m of these enzymes for BK is higher than that of ACE [2]. Their relative importance in the metabolism of BK in various biological milieus depends on their tissue distribution but also on the experimental conditions. Moreover, their capability to metabolize des-Arg^9-BK has often been overlooked.

    The role of ACE in the metabolism of BK has been studied in serum, in several tissues, namely the kidney [28], lung [29], skeletal muscle [30], and also in various types of cultured cells (synovial fibroblasts [31], endothelial cells [32] and vascular smooth muscle cells [33]). As the hypothetical role of endogenous BK and/or des-Arg^9-BK in the beneficial or side effects of ACEi is of considerable interest, we will focus on the kininase II function of ACE and the influence of its inhibition on the metabolism of kinins in blood and the cardiovascular system.

Role of ACE and influence of ACE inhibitors on the blood metabolism of kinins

Several authors have documented the metabolism of BK in serum and assessed the contribution of ACE to this process using serum from different animal species [2, 19, 22, 34, 35]. The degradation half-life ($t_{1/2}$) of BK and the relative importance of ACE have been evaluated using micromolar concentrations of BK added to blood fractions; such concentrations are superior to the K_m value of the ACE for BK and were necessary to allow detection of residual BK with HPLC separation and optical detection or bioassay.

Recently, the development of highly specific and sensitive chemiluminescent enzyme immunoassays for the quantification of BK and des-Arg^9-BK [36, 37] allowed the parallel exploration of the metabolism of both B_1 and B_2 agonists incubated at nanomolar concentrations in serum. This concentration range is believed to be more representative of the autocrine or paracrine production of endogenous kinins, as opposed to the micromolar concentrations used previously. Under these experimental conditions, Décarie et al. [38] reported a $t_{1/2}$ of 50 s when BK was incubated in presence of human serum, and even smaller values for rabbit, dog and rat serum, the animal species most used in the laboratory to investigate ACEi modulation of BK metabolism. In human serum, the rate of metabolism of des-Arg^9-BK (mean value 325 s) was similar to that measured for rabbit and dog but higher than that of rat serum (mean value 96 s). The same authors have also shown that ACE is the main metabolic pathway in this milieu, accounting for at least 50% of the degradation of BK. In human serum, they have estimated that ACE accounts for $76.0 \pm 7.5\%$ of the total enzyme activity responsible for the metabolism of BK. Two other enzymes account for the balance: kininase I (a minor metabolic pathway) and a third enzyme that we have recently identified as aminopeptidase P (APP) [39]. Des-Arg^9-BK is hydrolyzed by only two enzymes which also participate in the metabolism of BK: ACE and APP. In this case, however, APP represents the major and ACE the minor pathways for des-Arg^9-BK hydrolysis in serum.

The relative importance of ACE in the blood metabolism of kinins explain why complete *in vitro* inhibition of ACE with an ACEi increases significantly the $t_{1/2}$ of BK, this potentiating effect being more important than that measured for des-Arg^9-BK. However, ACE inhibition does not totally prevent the degradation of either peptide.

In 1990, Rigat et al. [40] described an insertion/deletion (I/D) polymorphism in the intron 16 of the ACE gene that accounts for 40% of the inter-individual variation in serum ACE activity. Recently, using a similar experimental approach [38], Brown et al. [41] were able to correlate the BK $t_{1/2}$ with the genotype of ACE. Individuals who were homozygous for the I allele and who exhibited the lowest activity of ACE also exhibited a significantly higher $t_{1/2}$ of BK when compared with the DD homozygous patients, who have a higher circulating ACE activity (*ex vivo* measurements in serum). These observations may be important for two reasons. Firstly, the D allele has been identified as an independent risk factor for myocardial infarction, left ventricular hypertrophy and progressive diabetic nephropathy [42–44]. Not only an increased transformation of AI into AII, but also a higher degradation of BK could be responsible, at least in part, for such diseases or complications. More recently, it has been reported that physical exercise performances are related with the ACE genotype, higher endurance being associated with the II genotype of the ACE gene [45]. BK could also be involved, at least in part, in this higher endurance. In fact, increased blood BK has been measured in the postexercise period [46].

Effect of ACE and ACE inhibitors on the metabolism of BK in the endothelium

As BK produces vasorelaxation via the endothelial release of NO, PGs and endothelium-derived hyperpolarizing factor, various approaches have been used to define the contribution of ACE and the influence of ACEi on the endothelial metabolism of BK. Grafe et al. [32] demonstrated that the metabolism of exogenous BK by endothelial cells was decreased when these cells were preincubated in the presence of an ACEi. At the endothelium level, Yamada et al. [47] have reported an important ACE labeling in the coronary vessels using quantitative autoradiography. More recently, Dumoulin et al. [48] have defined the metabolism of BK and the participation of ACE following a single passage through the coronary bed of isolated rat hearts. For this purpose, they perfused 10 ng/ml of BK in isolated hearts mounted according to Langendorff. They observed that the metabolism of BK is dependent on the perfusion rate, being more extensive for a low flow rate (1 ml/min) close to a level that produces ischemia. At the same flow rate, they were able to show an important participation of ACE in the metabolism of BK. Indeed, coperfusion of BK with an ACEi increased significantly (50%) the recovery of the native peptide and decreased the metabolism assessed by the degradation rate. However, ACE is not the sole enzyme responsible for the metabolism of BK in this experimental model. Neutral endopeptidase 24.11 (NEP) also contributes to the degradation of BK, but its role became significant only after ACE inhibition. Once again, these results are dependent on the experimental conditions, as the relative affinity of both enzymes for BK varied widely.

More recently, using the same experimental approach, it was shown for the first time that a chronic *in vivo* treatment with a dual peptidase inhibitor (omapatrilat) decreases also BK degradation by rat hearts [49]. Omapatrilat simultaneously inhibits ACE and NEP with a similar nanomolar affinity [50] and was used at 1 mg/kg per day, a dose previously reported to be hypotensive [51]. The inhibitory effect of a chronic simultaneous inhibition of ACE and NEP on BK degradation was greater than that of the simple ACE inhibition.

Metabolism of BK in the heart

ACE activity has been identified in membranes of vascular smooth muscle cells [33] and skeletal muscle cells [30] and its role in the metabolism of BK has been defined. However, the metabolism of BK at the level of cardiomyocytes is not well documented, although the benefical effect of ACEi has been demonstrated in acute and chronic cardiac pathologies. The contribution of ACE to the cardiac metabolism of BK was recently studied in normal, infarcted and hypertrophic rat hearts [52, 53]. For this purpose, membranes were prepared from hearts using an approach formerly described to define the role of ACE in the transformation of AI into AII [54]. This preparation, consisting of 75% cardiomyocyte membranes, is representative of the cardiac muscle [55]. As for the cited study based on serum [38], the interspecies differences in the metabolism of BK was studied. A major participation of ACE in the degradation of the peptide was observed (72.2% of the total kininase activity in normal human atria). These experiments confirm that ACE is a transmembrane enzyme not only at the endothelium, but also at the cardiomyocyte level. However, important interspecies differences in the metabolism of BK and in the effect of ACE inhibition on this metabolism could explain some discrepancies regarding the contribution of BK to the pharmacological effects of ACEi in different animal models.

Although ACEi therapy is largely used in the treatment of acute and chronic cardiac diseases, the influence of acute myocardial infarction (MI), remodeling and left ventricular hypertrophy on the degradation of BK was not defined until recently. The rat postinfarction model was used to define not only the effect of acute MI, but also of the chronic remodeling on the metabolism of BK [53]. This model has been widely used to study the pathophysiological processes involved in the acute and chronic postinfarction left ventricular remodeling. MI significantly shortens the $t_{1/2}$ of BK. In the infarcted zone, this decrease was established four days postinfarction and persists at least through day 35. In the noninfarcted portions of the MI hearts, BK $t_{1/2}$ also decreased significantly. The preincubation of membrane preparation with an ACEi increased the BK $t_{1/2}$, but the effect of ACEi varied as a function of the nature of the tissue (infarcted vs noninfarcted) and of the time of heart sampling. Indeed, in the early postinfarction period, ACEi did not normalize $t_{1/2}$, but its effect was evident 35 days post-MI; at a time where hypertrophy of the remaining myocardium was established. These observations show clearly that ACE is not the unique enzyme responsible for the inactivation of BK, although clearly important in that respect. Preincubation of the membranes with omapatrilat, the dual inhibitor of ACE and NEP, further increased BK $t_{1/2}$. The simultaneous inhibition of ACE and NEP was particularly effective one day post-MI. At that time, the participation of NEP in the degradation of BK equaled that of ACE. These *in vitro* observations will be the basis of further studies on the role of endogenous kinins in the acute and chronic postinfarction setting.

ACE, ACE inhibitors and B_2 receptors

Experimental evidence now exists for a cross-talk between ACE and B_2 receptors [56, 57]. These recent and interesting observations have been discussed elsewhere in this book.

ACE, ACE inhibitors and endogenous kinins

ACEi have been shown to be valuable therapeutic agents for the management of hypertension particularly with concomitant left ventricular hypertrophy, management of MI, chronic heart failure and diabetic nephropathy. These beneficial effects have been attributed to the inhibition of the formation of AII, a potent vasoconstrictor with growth factor-like effects, and to the inhibition of the metabolism of BK and potentiation of its antiproliferative and vasodilator effects [58–63]. The significance of the kinin receptor subtype duality (B_1, B_2) and the relative importance of individual endogenous kinins (BK, des-Arg^9-BK and homologue peptides) are largely unexplored issues in the analysis of the beneficial and side effects of ACEi at the present time.

Endogenous kinins and the beneficial effect of ACE inhibitors: pharmacological evidence

The rationale supporting the participation of kinins (mainly BK) in the therapeutic effects of ACEi has been extensively reviewed [60]. The evaluation of the contribution of BK to the cardiovascular effect of ACEi is largely based on pharmacological evidence. In various experimental animals, the effects of ACEi are similar to those of BK and are blocked by icatibant (Hoe 140; an antagonist of the preformed B_2 receptors). These observations have been made both *in vivo* and *in vitro*, suggesting the presence of an intriguing multi-component KKS in some cultured cells or isolated tissues. In endothelial cells cultured in the presence of an ACEi, Wiemer et al. [61, 62] have shown an increased production of NO and PGI$_2$, mediators typically released by BK. Preincubation of the cells with icatibant decreased the secretory effect of ACEi. *In vivo* the potential role of BK in the antihypertensive, antiproliferative and antihypertrophic effects of ACEi has been investigated using chronic treatment with icatibant [64]. Some of these results are conflicting and may be affected by the precise experimental conditions. As far as the animal models are concerned, it is remarkable that the hypotensive effect of ACEi in the rat during by B_2 receptor blockade by icatibant varies depending on the model. In a renovascular model of hypertension in the Wistar rat (two kidneys, one clip), about one third of the therapeutic effect of an ACEi was reversed by icatibant [59]; the latter antagonist peptide did not influence the therapeutic effect of ramipril in spontaneously hypertensive rats, a genetically determined pathology [59]. In contrast, the acute hypotensive effect of captopril is entirely abrogated by icatibant in a model where rats are pretreated with deoxycorticosterone acetate and high salt intake (a model of primary hyperaldosteronism with high urinary kallikrein) [64]. Similar results were also obtained in a limited number of normotensive and hypertensive patients; the short-term decrease of mean arterial pressure induced by captopril was significantly attenuated by injection of icatibant [65]. Most hypertensive humans do not suffer from the renovascular or endocrine forms of the disease and patients with essential hypertension exhibit normal, or even low, urinary kallikrein [66] suggesting that their renal KKS is not overtly activated. Moreover, B_1 receptor antagonists have not been exploited so far in the analysis of kinin contribution to ACEi actions; *per se*, treatment of normal rabbits with high doses of ACEi did not induce B_1 receptors (mRNA in hearts and functional hemodynamic responses [67]), but the effect of hypertension, with or without end organ damage, on B_1 receptor expression in tissues has not yet been well documented.

The participation of BK in the protective effect of ACEi during the ischemia-reperfusion has also been studied *in vitro* using isolated perfused heart. The results varied according to the experimental model. ACEi and BK perfusion have been shown to have similar if not identical effects: decreased cardiac enzyme release into the effluent, preservation of ATP stores and decreased incidence of arrhythmia [68]; these effects being prevented by coperfusion of icatibant. In a similar model of perfused heart, other authors [69] have observed that des-Arg^9-BK, but not BK, decreased the arrhythmia incidence during reperfusion, this effect being inhibited by coperfusion of the B_1 receptor antagonist, Lys-[Leu^8]-des-Arg^9-BK, but not by a B_2 receptor antagonist.

Effect of ACE blockade on endogenous kinins

Effect of ACE inhibitors on endogenous kinins in cultured cells
Using cultured bovine aortic endothelial cells, Wiemer and Wirth [70] were able to measure immunoreactive kinin in the supernatant at an average concentration of 100 pg/ml. Preincubation with ramiprilat (10^{-8} M) significantly increased by five-fold the concentration of the immunoreactive material. This preservative effect of ACEi on the immunoreactive BK measured in the culture supernatant has complemented the previous observations on the potentiating effect of ACEi on the second messenger of the B_2 agonist.

A similar potentiating effect of ACEi could be measured on the release of immunoreactive BK by rat cardiac myocytes. In this model, cilazaprilat (10^{-5} M) significantly increased by 4.5 times the immunoreactive BK measured in the culture medium after a 5.5 h hypoxemia [11]. This protective effect of ACE inhibition on the B_2 agonist was negatively related to the release of CK. Under the same experimental conditions, BK production could not be observed for nonmyocytic cardiac cells [11].

Effect of ACE inhibitors on endogenous kinins in experimental ischemia-reperfusion models

In *in vitro* model of heart ischemia, immunoreactive kinins could be detected in the cardiac effluent at the reperfusion. The concentration of the immunoreactive kinin measured (ng vs pg) and the nature of the potentiating effect of the ACEi reported (only on BK or on BK and des-Arg^9-BK) were furthermore conflicting [71, 72]. More recently, and for the first time, we observed that a chronic treatment with an ACEi or the vasopeptidase inhibitor omapatrilat potentiates the release of endogenous BK in the effluent after a total *in vitro* ischemia of rat heart. (A. Adam et al., unpublished observation).

Effect of ACE inhibitors on tissue kinins in experimental models

The effect of chronic or acute treatment with an ACEi on the tissue content of endogenous kinins has been studied in different models. Campbell et al. [73] have shown that a chronic treatment with an ACEi potentiated the BK content in different tissues such as kidney, heart and lung. This increase depended on the dose of the ACEi. In heart of rats sacrificed 26 days post-MI induced by a coronary artery ligation, the same authors [74] could not measure a similar potentiating effect of a chronic treatment with an ACEi on the heart content of BK. They could, however, observe a significant reduction in the tissue AII/AI ratio and an inhibition of the cardiac hypertrophy.

In a model of acute inflammation induced locally by injection of carrageenan, a coinjection or a chronic treatment with an ACEi potentiates the local content of both BK and des-Arg^9-BK at the local inflammatory site confirming that ACE is responsible for the metabolism of both kinins. In this experimental model, however, only BK was involved in the local inflammatory process [36, 75].

Effect of ACE blockade on blood immunoreactive kinins in humans

The sampling of venous blood, the one readily available in clinical settings, or of urine are far from ideal to assess possible drug-induced BK potentiation. Careful analysis of the papers that offer the best methodological approaches reveal that BK or des-Arg^9-BK concentrations are not significantly increased in the venous blood of patients under pharmacological ACE blockade. In venous blood sampled in normal humans, the average concentration of immunoreactive des-Arg^9-BK (204 pg/ml) is higher than that of BK (67 pg/ml) [76]. Despite the fact that the kininase I activity is a minor metabolic pathway for BK, the $t_{1/2}$ for des-Arg^9-BK is comparatively so large that the latter peptide apparently accumulates. These values are not significantly changed in patients with essential hypertension or under ACE blockade with enalapril. The urine of these subjects also contains both BK and des-Arg^9-BK immunoreactivities that do not differ between groups [76]. The authors point out that venous blood measurements may not reflect the status of the kinins at the tissue level, owing to metabolism by multiple pathways. Patients with renal failure exhibit plasma BK and des-Arg^9-BK concentrations similar to those reported in normal patients, the des-Arg^9-BK immunoreactivity being larger than that of BK [77]. Again, ACE blockade failed to modify these levels. Another recent study with a different design (paired measurement before and after the oral administration of quinapril in normal volunteers) allowed the measurement of a significant, but rather small, increase in venous blood BK concentration [78]. Whether BK concentration in peripheral vascular tissue differs from the venous blood level and is more affected by ACEi is an important issue that may limit the significance of the blood concentrations of kinins.

Endogenous kinins and the side effects of ACE inhibitors

The most frequent side effect associated with chronic ACEi administration is a nonproductive cough that has been hypothetically attributed to the accumulation of endogenous BK. This mediator has also been considered as being responsible of three other types of ACEi side effects: angioedema (AO), anaphylactoid reactions (AR) in hemodialysis and severe hypotensive reaction (SHR) during blood product transfusion. Until now, there is no clinical evidence that directly implicates endogenous BK in cough. In guinea pigs, captopril greatly exaggerated the cough reaction to inhaled citric acid (a standard tussigenic stimulus), and this effect of captopril was prevented by icatibant [79]. Only one group has recently reported some evidence for an increase in BK during acute drug-induced angioedema [80].

Increased blood levels of BK have been reported *in vitro* and *in vivo* in patients and in animals experiencing anaphylactoid reactions during hemodialysis with a negatively charged dialysis membrane in the presence of an ACEi [81–83]. To address the pathophysiological background of the side effects of ACEi, we have analyzed the metabolism of BK and des-Arg^9-BK in the serum of patients who experienced severe reactions that could be attributed to kinins. We were not able to show any difference in the metabolism of BK, as compared to healthy control patients, but that of des-Arg^9-BK was a more fruitful area of investigation. Indeed, des-Arg^9-BK exhibited an increased $t_{1/2}$ of degradation in patients with associated AO [84], AR [39] and SHR [85]. This parameter was still abnormal when serum samples were preincubated in the presence of an ACEi. Moreover, when ACE was completely inhibited *in vitro*, neither the nature or the concentration of ACEi influenced the metabolism of either B_1 or B_2 agonist. The increased $t_{1/2}$ of des-Arg^9-BK could be negatively correlated with the enzyme activity of aminopeptidase P (APP) [39, 86], the main enzyme found responsible for the metabolism of des-Arg^9-BK [39].

Conclusion

BK and des-Arg^9-BK are natural substrates for ACE. ACEi have been shown
to protect both peptides against their *in vitro* metabolism in various experimental models. *In vitro*, BK and des-Arg^9-BK reproduce some pharmacological effects of ACEi. Many experimental systems support, to various extents,
the role of BK and/or des-Arg^9-BK in the pharmacological effects of ACEi.
However, at the present time, strong causal and direct evidence of the mediation of ACEi actions by endogenous BK and/or des-Arg^9-BK is still missing.
The same gap exists for the analysis of some side effects of ACEi. In the case
of the therapeutic effects, it is not clear whether beneficial vasodilator effects
of endogenous kinins can be dissociated from their inflammatory actions.
However, several end points of ACEi action convey the concept of tissue injury
and inflammation (ischemia, infarction, tissue remodeling) and represent situations where the inflammatory nature of kinins can be reconciled with cardiovascular physiopathology and where both kinin receptors and kininase gene
expression could be locally modulated. The understanding of the contribution
of ACE, but also that of NEP and other enzymes, to the metabolism of BK constitutes a prerequisite to elucidate the importance of endogenous kinins in the
cardioprotective effects of ACEi.

References

1 Bhoola KD, Figueroa CD, Worthy K (1992) Bioregulation of kinins: kallikreins, kininogens and
   kininases. *Pharmacol Rev* 44: 1–80
2 Erdös EG, Skidgel RA (1997) Metabolism of bradykinin by peptidases in health and disease. *In*:
   SG Farmer (ed.): *The Kinin System*. Academic Press, San Diego, 111–141
3 Marceau F (1995) Kinin B$_1$ receptors: a review. *Immunopharmacology* 30: 1–26
4 Marceau F, Hess JF, Bachvarov DR (1998) The B$_1$ receptors for kinins. *Pharmacol Rev* 50:
   357–386
5 Auch-Schwelk W, Kuchenbuch C, Walther CB, Bossaller C, Friedel N, Graf K, Grafe M, Fleck E
   (1993) Local regulation of vascular tone by bradykinin and angiotensin converting enzyme
   inhibitors. *Eur Heart J* 14 (suppl I): 154–160
6 Mombouli JV, Vanhoutte PM (1995) Kinins and endothelial control of vascular smooth muscle.
   Annu Rev Pharmacol Toxicol 35: 679–705
7 Rioux F, Bachelard H, St-Pierre S, Barabé J (1987) Epicardial application of bradykinin elicits
   pressor effects and tachycardia in guinea pigs. Possible mechanisms. *Peptides* 8: 863–868
8 Nolly HL, Lima MC, Carretero OA, Scicli AG (1992) The kallikrein-kinin system in blood vessels. *Agents Actions Suppl* 38/III: 1–9
9 Nolly H, Carbini LA, Scicli G, Carretero O, Scicli AG (1994) A local kallikrein-kinin system is
   present in rat hearts. *Hypertension* 23: 919–923
10 Gräfe M, Bossaller C, Graf K, Auch-Schwelk W, Baumgarten CR, Hildebrandt A, Fleck E (1993)
   Effect of angiotensin-converting-enzyme inhibition on bradykinin metabolism by vascular
   endothelial cells. *Amer J Physiol* 264 (*Heart Circ Physiol* 33): H1493–H1497
11 Matoba S, Tatsumi T, Keira N, Kawahara A, Akashi K, Kobara M, Asayama J, Nakagawa M
   (1999) Cardioprotective effect of angiotensin-converting enzyme inhibition against
   hypoxia/reoxygenation injury in cultured rat cardiac myocytes. *Circulation* 99: 817–822
12 Ferreira SH, Vane JR (1967) The disappearance of bradykinin and eledoisin in the circulation and
   vascular beds of the cat. *Brit J Pharmacol Chemother* 30: 417–424
13 Ferreira SH (1965) A bradykinin-potentiating factor (BPF) present in the venom of *Bothrops*

jararaca. Brit J Pharmacol Chemother 24: 163–169

14 Bakhle YS (1968) Conversion of angiotensin I to angiotensin II by cell-free extracts of dog lung. *Nature* 220: 919–921

15 Ng KKF, Vane JR (1968) Fate of angiotensin I in the circulation. *Nature* 218: 144–150

16 Cushman DW, Ondetti MA (1980) Inhibitors of angiotensin-converting enzyme. *Prog Med Chem* 17: 42–104

17 Dorer FE, Kahn JR, Lentz KE, Levine M, Skeggs LT (1974) Hydrolysis of bradykinin by angiotensin-converting enzyme. *Circ Res* 34: 824–827

18 Dorer FE, Ryan JW, Steward JM (1974) Hydrolysis of bradykinin and its higher homologues by angiotensin-converting enzyme. *Biochem J* 141: 915–917

19 Sheikh IA, Kaplan AP (1986) Studies of the digestion of bradykinin, Lys-bradykinin and desArg^9-bradykinin by angiotensin converting enzyme. *Biochem Pharmacol* 35: 1951–1956

20 Bunning P, Riordan JF (1983) Activation of angiotensin converting enzyme by monovalent anions. *Biochemistry* 22: 110–116

21 Bunning P, Holmquist B, Riordan JF (1983) Substrate specificity and kinetic characteristics of angiotensin converting enzyme. *Biochemistry* 22: 103–110

22 Drapeau G, Chow A, Ward PE (1991) Metabolism of bradykinin analogs by angiotensin I converting enzyme and carboxypeptidase N. *Peptides* 12: 631–638

23 Oshima G, Hiraga Y, Shirono K, Oh-ishi S, Sakakibara S, Kinoshita T (1985) Cleavage of des-Arg^9-bradykinin by angiotensin I-converting enzyme from pig kidney cortex. *Experientia* 41: 325–328

24 Cheung HS, Wang FL, Ondetti MA, Sabo EF, Cushman DW (1980) Binding of peptide substrates and inhibitors of angiotensin-converting enzyme. Importance of the COOH-terminal dipeptide sequence. *J Biol Chem* 255: 401–407

25 Erdös EG, Skidgel RA (1985) Structure and functions of human angiotensin I converting enzyme (kininase II). *Biochem Soc Trans* 13: 42–44

26 Jaspard E, Wei L, Alhenc-Gelas F (1993) Differences in the properties and enzymatic specificities of the two active sites of angiotensin I-converting enzyme (kininase II). *J Biol Chem* 268: 9496–9503

27 Jaspard E, Alhenc-Gelas F (1995) Catalytic properties of the two active sites of angiotensin I-converting enzyme on the cell surface. *Biochem Biophys Res Commun* 211: 528–534

28 Ura N, Carretero OA, Erdös EG (1987) Role of renal endopeptidase 24.11 in kinin metabolism *in vitro* and *in vivo*. *Kidney Int* 32: 507–513

29 Dragovic T, Igic R, Erdös EG, Rabito SF (1993) Metabolism of bradykinin by peptidases in the lung. *Amer Rev Respir Dis* 147: 1491–1496

30 Ward PE, Russell JS, Vaghy PL (1995) Angiotensin and bradykinin metabolism by peptidases identified in skeletal muscle. *Peptides* 16: 1073–1078

31 Bathon JM, Proud D, Mizutani S, Ward PE (1992) Cultured human synovial fibroblasts rapidly metabolize kinins and neuropeptides. *J Clin Invest* 90: 981–991

32 Graf K, Gräfe M, Auch-Schwelk W, Baumgarten CR, Bossaller C, Fleck E (1992) Bradykinin degrading activity in cultured human endothelial cells. *J Cardiovasc Pharmacol* 20 (suppl 9): S16–S20

33 Mentlein R, Roos T (1996) Proteases involved in the metabolism of angiotensin II, bradykinin, calcitonin-gene related peptide (CGRP) and neuropeptide Y by vascular muscle cells. *Peptides* 17: 709–720

34 Marceau F, Gendreau M, Barabé J, St-Pierre S, Regoli D (1981) The degradation of bradykinin (BK) and des-Arg^9-BK in plasma. *Can J Physiol Pharmacol* 59: 131–138

35 Ishida H, Scicli AG, Carretero OA (1989) Contributions of various rat plasma peptidases to kinin hydrolysis. *J Pharmacol Exp Ther* 251: 817–820

36 Décarie A, Drapeau G, Closset J, Couture R, Adam A (1994) Development of digoxigenin-labeled peptide: application to chemiluminoenzyme immunoassay of bradykinin in inflamed tissues. *Peptides* 15: 511–518

37 Raymond P, Drapeau G, Raut R, Audet R, Marceau F, Ong H, Adam A (1995) Quantification of des-Arg^9-bradykinin using a chemiluminescence enzyme immunoassay: application to its kinetic profile during plasma activation. *J Immunol Method* 180: 247–257

38 Décarie A, Raymond P, Gervais N, Couture R, Adam A (1996) Serum interspecies differences in metabolic pathways of bradykinin and des-Arg^9-BK: influence of enalaprilat. *Amer J Physiol* 270 (*Heart Circ Physiol* 39): H1340–H1347

39 Blais CJr Marc-Aurèle J, Simmons WH, Loute G, Thibault P, Skidgel R, Adam A (1999) Des-Arg^9-bradykinin metabolism in patients who presented hypersensitivity reactions during hemodialysis: role of serum ACE and aminopeptidase P. *Peptides* 20: 421–430
40 Rigat B, Hubert C, Alhenc-Gelas F, Cambien F, Corvol P, Soubrier F (1990) An insertion/deletion polymorphism in the angiotensin I-converting enzyme gene accounting for half of the variance of serum enzyme levels. *J Clin Invest* 86: 1343–1346
41 Brown NJ, Blais CJr Gandhi SK, Adam A (1998) ACE insertion/deletion genotype affects bradykinin metabolism. *J Cardiovasc Pharmacol* 32: 373–377
42 Cambien F, Poirier O, Lecerf L, Evans A, Cambou JP, Arveiler D, Luc G, Bard JM, Bara L, Ricard S et al (1992) Deletion polymorphism in the gene for angiotensin-converting enzyme is a potent risk factor for myocardial infarction. *Nature* 359: 641–644
43 Schunkert H, Hense HW, Holmer SR, Stender K, Perz S, Keil U, Lorell BH, Riegger GAJ (1994) Association between a deletion polymorphism of the angiotensin-converting-enzyme gene and left ventricular hypertrophy. *N Engl J Med* 330: 1634–1648
44 Marre M, Bernardet P, Gallois Y, Savagner G, Guyene TT, Hallab M, Cambien F, Passa P, Alhenc-Gelas F (1994) Relationships between angiotensin I-converting enzyme gene polymorphism, plasma levels, and diabetic retinal and renal complications. *Diabetes* 43: 384–388
45 Montgomery HE, Marshall R, Hemingway H, Myerson S (1998) Human gene for physical performance. *Science* 193: 221
46 Blais CJr Adam A, Massicote D, Peronnet F (1999) Increase in blood bradykinin concentration following eccentric weight-training exercise in man. *J Appl Physiol* 87 (3): 163–172
47 Yamada H, Fabris B, Allen AM, Jackson CI, Mendelsohn AO (1991) Localization of angiotensin converting enzyme in rat heart. *Circ Res* 68: 141–149
48 Dumoulin MJ, Adam A, Blais CJr Lamontagne D (1998) Metabolism of bradykinin by the coronary vascular bed. *Cardiovasc Res* 38: 229–236
49 Dumoulin MJ, Adam A, Rouleau JL, Lamontagne D (2001) Comparison of omapatrilat with NEP and ACE inhibition on bradykinin metabolism in the coronary vascular bed. *J Cardiovasc Pharmacol* 37: 359–366
50 Trippodo NC, Fox M, Natarajan V, Panchal BC, Dorso CR, Asaad MM (1993) Combined inhibition of neutral endopeptidase and angiotensin converting enzyme in cardiomyopathic hamsters with compensated heart failure. *J Pharmacol Exp Ther* 267: 108–116
51 Liu YH, Yang XP, Sharov VG, Nass O, Peterson HN, Carretero OA (1997) Effects of angiotensin-converting enzyme inhibitors and angiotensin II type 1 receptor antagonists in rats with heart failure. Role of kinins and angiotensin II type 2 receptors. *J Clin Invest* 99: 1926–1935
52 Blais CJr Drapeau G, Raymond P, Lamontagne D, Gervais N, Venneman I, Adam A (1997) Contribution of angiotensin-converting enzyme to the cardiac metabolism of bradykinin: an interspecies study. *Amer J Physiol* 273 (*Heart Circ Physiol* 42): H2263–H2271
53 Raut R, Rouleau JL, Blais CJr Gosselin H, Molinaro G, Sirois MG, Lepage Y, Crine P, Adam A (1999) Bradykinin metabolism in the postinfarcted rat heart: role of ACE and neutral endopeptidase 24.11. *Amer J Physiol* 276 (*Heart Circ Physiol* 45): H1769–H1779
54 Kinoshita AH, Urata H, Bumpus FM, Husain A (1993) Measurement of angiotensin I converting enzyme inhibition in the heart. *Circ Res* 73: 51–60
55 Weber KT, Brilla CG (1991) Pathological hypertrophy and cardiac interstitium: fibrosis and renin-angiotensin-aldosterone system. *Circulation* 83: 1849–1865
56 Minshall RD, Erdös EG, Vogel SM (1997) Angiotensin I-converting enzyme inhibitors potentiate bradykinin's inotropic effects independently of blocking its activation. *Amer J Cardiol* 80 (suppl 3A): 132A–136A
57 Minshall RD, Tan F, Nakamura F, Rabito SF, Becker RP, Marcic B, Erdös EG (1997) Potentiation of the actions of bradykinin by angiotensin I-converting enzyme inhibitors. The role of expressed human bradykinin B$_2$ receptors and angiotensin I-converting enzyme in CHO cells. *Circ Res* 81: 848–856
58 Unger T, Gohlke P, Gruber MG (1990) Converting enzyme inhibitors. *In*: D Ganten, PJ Murlow (eds): *Handbook of Experimental Pharmacology*. Vol 3. Springer Verlag, Berlin/Heidelberg, 110–116
59 Unger T, Gohlke P (1994) Converting enzyme inhibitors in cardiovascular therapy: current status and future potential. *Cardiovasc Res* 28: 146–158
60 Linz W, Wiemer G, Gohlke P, Unger T, Schölkens BA (1995) Contribution of kinins to the cardiovascular actions of angiotensin-converting enzyme inhibitors. *Pharmacol Rev* 47: 25–49

61 Wiemer G, Popp R, Schölkens BA, Gogelein H (1994) Enhancement of cytosolic calcium, prostacyclin and nitric oxyde by bradykinin and the ACE inhibitor ramiprilat in porcine brain capillary endothelial cells. *Brain Res* 638: 261–266

62 Wiemer G, Schölkens BA, Linz W (1994) Endothelial protection by converting enzyme inhibitors. *Cardiovasc Res* 28: 166–172

63 Farhy RD, Carretero OA, Ho KL, Scicli AG (1993) Role of kinins and nitric oxide in the effects of angiotensin converting enzyme inhibitors on neointima formation. *Circ Res* 72: 1202–1210

64 Chen K, Zhang X, Dunham EW, Zimmerman BG (1996) Kinin-mediated antihypertensive effect of captopril in deoxycorticosterone acetate-salt hypertension. *Hypertension* 27: 85–89

65 Gainer JV, Morrow JD, Loveland A, King DJ, Brown NJ (1998) Effect of bradykinin receptor blockade on the response to angiotensin-converting-enzyme inhibitor in normotensive and hypertensive subjects. *N Engl J Med* 339: 1285–1292

66 Margolius HS, Horwitz D, Geller RG, Alexander RW, Gill JR, Pisano JJ, Keiser HR (1974) Urinary kallikrein excretion in hypertensive man: relationship to sodium intake and sodium retaining steroids. *Circ Res* 35: 820–825

67 Marceau F, Larrivée JF, Saint-Jacques E, Bachvarov DR (1997) The kinin B_1 receptor: an inducible G protein coupled receptor. *Can J Physiol Pharmacol* 75: 725–730

68 Linz W, Martorana PA, Schölkens BA (1990) Local inhibition of bradykinin degradation in ischemic hearts. *J Cardiovasc Pharmacol* 15 (suppl 6): S99–S109

69 Chahine R, Adam A, Yamaguchi N, Gaspo R, Regoli D, Nadeau R (1993) Protective effects of bradykinin on the ischemic heart: implication of the B_1 receptor. *Brit J Pharmacol* 108: 318–322

70 Wiemer G, Wirth K (1992) Production of cyclic GMP via activation of B_1 and B_2 kinin receptors in cultured bovine aortic endothelial cells. *J Pharmacol Exp Ther* 262: 729–733

71 Baumgarten CR, Linz W, Kunkel G, Schölkens BA, Wiemer G (1993) Ramiprilat increases bradykinin outflow from isolated rat hearts. *Brit J Pharmacol* 108: 293–295

72 Lamontagne D, Nadeau R, Adam A (1995) Effect of enalaprilat on bradykinin and des-Arg^9-bradykinin release following reperfusion of the ischaemic rat heart. *Brit J Pharmacol* 115: 476–478

73 Campbell DJ, Kladis A, Duncan AM (1993) Effects of converting enzyme inhibitors on angiotensin and bradykinin peptides. *Hypertension* 23: 439–449

74 Duncan AM, Burrell LM, Kladis A, Campbell DJ (1996) Effects of angiotensin-converting enzyme inhibition on angiotensin and bradykinin peptides in rats with myocardial infarction. *J Cardiovasc Pharmacol* 28: 746–754

75 Décarie A, Adam A, Couture R (1996) Effects of captopril and icatibant on bradykinin (BK) and des[Arg^9]BK in carrageenan induced edema. *Peptides* 17: 1009–1015

76 Odya CE, Wilgis FP, Walker JF, Oparil S (1983) Immunoreactive bradykinin and [des-Arg^9]-bradykinin in low-renin essential hypertension before and after treatment with enalapril (MK 421). *J Lab Clin Med* 102: 714–721

77 Marceau F, Brochu S, Pelletier I, Drapeau G, Adam A, Lebel M (1995) Inflammatory peptides at the beginning of hemodialysis in asymptomatic patients treated or not with angiotensin I-converting inhibitors. *Nephron* 71: 474–476

78 Pellacani A, Brunner HR, Nussberger J (1994) Plasma kinins increase after angiotensin- converting enzyme inhibition in human subjects. *Clin Sci* 87: 567–574

79 Fox AJ, Lalloo UG, Belvisi MG, Bernareggi M, Chung KF, Barnes PJ (1996) Bradykinin-evoked sensitization of airway sensory nerves: a mechanism for ACE–inhibitor cough. *Nat Med* 2: 814–817

80 Nussberger J, Cugno M, Amstutz C, Cicardi M, Pellacani A, Agostoni A (1998) Plasma bradykinin in angiooedema. *Lancet* 351: 1693–1697

81 Renaux J-L, Thomas M, Crost T, Loughraeib N, Vantard G (1999) Activation of the kallikrein-kinin system in hemodialysis: role of membrane electronegativity, blood dilution and pH. *Kidney Int* 55: 1097–1103

82 Verresen L, Fink E, Lemke HD, Vanrenterghem Y (1994) Bradykinin is a mediator of anaphylactoid reactions during hemodialysis with AN69 membranes. *Kidney Int* 45: 1497–1503

83 Krieter DH, Grude M, Lemke HD, Fink E, Bonner G, Schölkens BA, Schulz E, Muller GA (1998) Anaphylactoid reactions during hemodialysis in sheep are ACE inhibitor dose-dependent and mediated by bradykinin. *Kidney Int* 53: 1026–1035

84 Blais CJr Rouleau JL, Brown NJ, Lepage Y, Spence D, Munoz C, Friborg J, Geadah D, Gervais N, Adam A (1999) Serum metabolism of bradykinin (BK) and des-Arg^9-BK in patients with ACE

inhibitor (ACEI)–associated angioedema (AE). *Immunopharmacology* 43: 293–302

85 Cyr M, Hume HA, Champagne M, Sweeney JD, Blais CJr Gervais N, Adam A (1999) Anomaly of the des-Arg^9-bradykinin metabolism associated with severe hypotensive reactions during blood transfusions: a preliminary study. *Transfusion* 39: 1084–1088

86 Prechel MM, Orawski AT, Maggiora LL, Simmons WH (1995) Effect of a new aminopeptidase P inhibitor, apstatin, on bradykinin degradation in the rat lung. *J Pharmacol Exp Ther* 275: 1136–1142

ACE Inhibitors
ed. by P. D'Orléans-Juste and G.E. Plante
© 2001 Birkhäuser Verlag/Switzerland

Role of the renin-angiotensin system on the central and peripheral autonomic nervous system

Jacques de Champlain[1] and Pedro D'Orléans-Juste[2]

[1] *Research Group on Autonomic Nervous System, Department of Physiology, Faculty of Medicine, Université de Montréal, Montréal (Quebec), Canada*
[2] *Department of Pharmacology, Faculty of Medicine, Université de Sherbrooke, Sherbrooke (Québec), Canada*

Introduction

The renin-angiotensin system (RAS) and the autonomic nervous system (ANS) play a major role in the maintenance of cardiovascular homeostasis. The RAS does not only influence the cardiovascular system through the endocrine role of the kidney RAS, but also through the paracrine actions of local RAS which have been demonstrated in various other organs such as the heart, vessels, brain and adrenal glands. On the other hand, the ANS is closely linked to the cardiovascular system by a dense network of sympathetic and parasympathetic nerves, as well as by the endocrine role of catecholamines released from the adrenal medulla. The activity of the ANS is controlled by the activity of afferent fibers derived from stretchreceptors, baroreceptors and chemoreceptors localized in the heart, large vessels and lungs which modulate and influence the baroreflex responses through the cardio and vasomotor centers localized in the hypothalamus and in the brain stem (Fig. 1).

Angiotensin II (AII) participates in the regulation of the cardiovascular system by its pressor effects resulting from various mechanisms such as its direct vasoconstrictor effect, the liberation of aldosterone and the regulation of the water and electrolyte balance, as well as through its central and peripheral facilitation of sympathetic activity. On the other hand, the participation of the sympathetic system in cardiovascular homeostasis results directly from the action of sympathetic neurotransmitters on their specific receptors, as well as indirectly through the activation of the RAS by stimulation of β-adrenoreceptors by noradrenaline (NA).

Most of the actions of AII are mediated through the AT_1 receptors which are coupled to membrane G proteins. The activation of the AT_1 receptor results in the hydrolysis of phosphoinositide as well as in the inhibition of adenylate cyclase. This receptor is involved in the acute hemodynamic response, as well as in the long-term growth stimulation of cardiac and vascular cells induced by AII. Because of its deleterious effects on the cardiovascular system, AII has

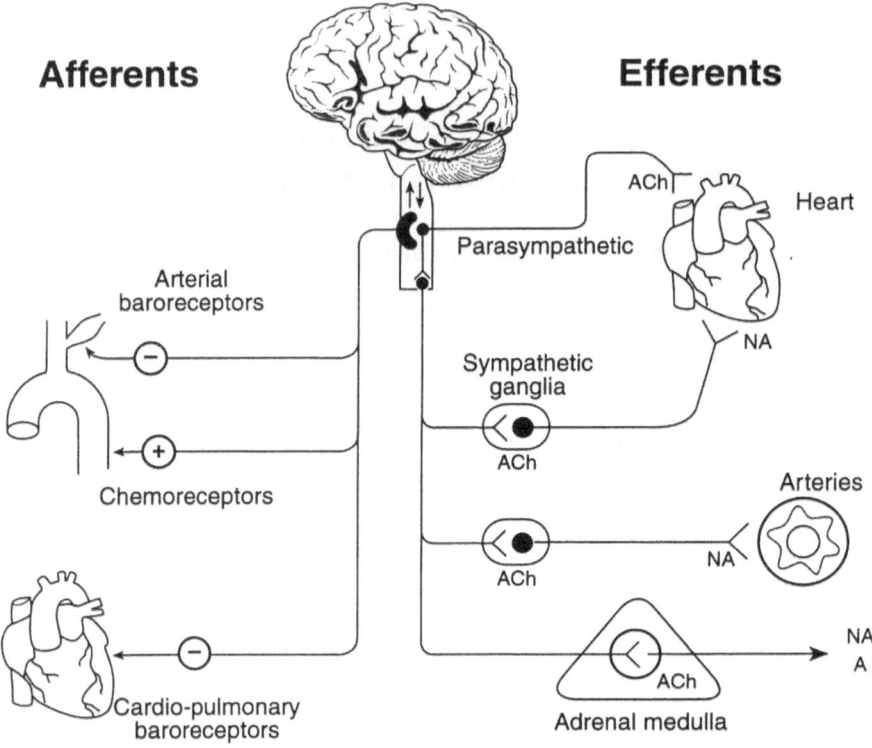

Figure 1. Afferent and efferent fibers of the autonomic nervous system and their influences on the cardiovascular system.

become a major target in the pharmacological treatment of hypertension and heart failure. Numerous angiotensin converting enzyme inhibitors (ACEI), as well as non-peptidic AT_1 blockers, have been developed to counteract the effects of the RAS on the cardiovascular system.

Although the etiology of essential hypertension is recognized to be multi-factorial, treatments with ACEI or AT_1 blockers have been shown efficacious in an important proportion of essential hypertensive patients. It thus appears that the RAS constitutes a major component of the interactive mechanism postulated to underly the development and maintenance of hypertension in humans. Since no correlations were demonstrated between circulating renin or angiotensin levels and the hypotensive effects of RAS blockade, this suggests that local RAS and/or interactions between RAS and other systems could play an important role in the maintenance of hypertension.

The ANS has also been postulated to play a major role in the development and maintenance of hypertension in experimental animal models as well as in humans [1]. An increase in the sympathetic tone and reactivity has been postulated in essential hypertension based on increased microneurographic recording intensity, increased NA spillover in the heart and kidney, as well as on increased circulating NA and adrenaline levels. Moreover, a reduction in the parasympathetic tone has also been documented in human hypertension. The numerous interactions which have been demonstrated between RAS and ANS could thus synergically contribute to the development and maintenance of hypertension in humans. Such mechanisms could explain the inhibition of the RAS by the blockade of β-adrenoceptors, as well as the sympatholitic effect of RAS blockade in human hypertension.

Interactions between the RAS and the sympathetic system may occur centrally at the level of vasomotor centers as well as in the periphery at the level of presynaptic and postsynaptic sympathetic mechanisms. Indeed, AII has been found to modulate the sensitivity of baroreflex mechanisms, to increase the centrally-controlled sympathetic system activity as well as to facilitate the neurotransmission at the level of sympathetic ganglia, peripheral sympathetic fibers and adrenal medulla [2]. In the periphery, the enhanced sympathetic neurotransmission can result from the inhibition of NA reuptake by sympathetic fibers, an enhanced catecholamine synthesis, a facilitation of NA liberation by the activation of AT_1 presynaptic receptors as well as by the increase in the sensitivity of postsynaptic vasoconstrictive adrenergic receptors [3] (Fig. 2). On the other hand, renin secretion by the kidney has been demonstrated to be neurally controlled by the sympathetic system [4] through the stimulation of β-adrenoceptors located on juxtaglomerular cells [5]. A similar renin-stimulatory mechanism has also been demonstrated *in vivo* in the human vascular RAS [6].

Modulation of central autonomic system by RAS

It is established that the sensitivity of baroreflex can be modulated by circulating hormones and by various neurotransmitters interacting at the level of vasomotor centers localized in the brain stem and hypothalamus [7]. In numerous experimental models of hypertension, as well as in human hypertension, it has been demonstrated that the sensitivity of the baroreflex is reset to respond at higher blood pressure levels [8]. The RAS could participate in this phenomenon since AII has been reported to inhibit centrally the negative feedback on efferent sympathetic activation of the heart during baroreceptor stimulation [9, 10]. Indeed it was found that the administration of AII attenuated the bradycardic response during a rise in blood pressure and potentiated the chronotropic response during a fall in blood pressure in normotensive conditions. The central action of AII could be mediated through the activation of the central sympathetic neurons in the rostro-ventrolateral medulla which innervates preganglionic neurons or else could be mediated through alterations of the afferences originating from the area prostrema. Moreover, it has been postulated that circulating AII levels originating from peripheral RAS could also contribute to the attenuation of baroreflex functions in spontaneously hypertensive

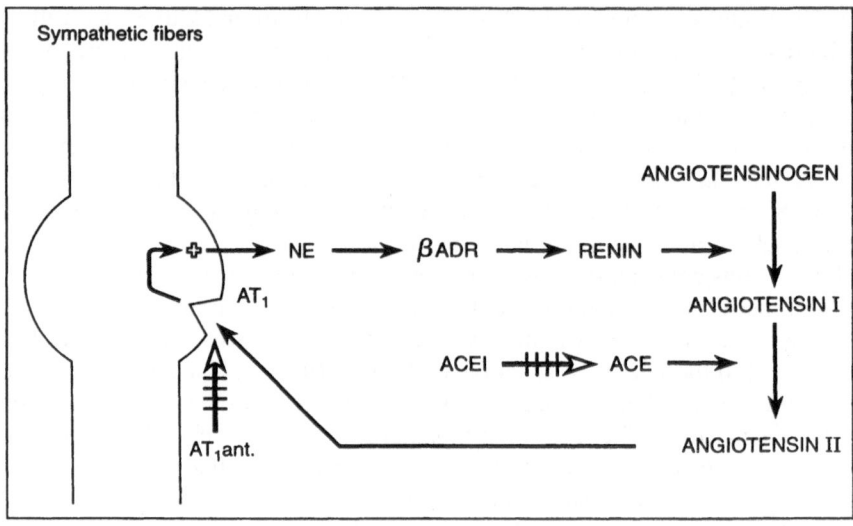

Figure 2. Angiotensin II modulates the neurotransmission at the level of the peripheral sympathetic fiber and consequently the renin-angiotensin pathway in the kidney.

rats (SHR) [12]. Since central regions where circulating AII levels can interact are richly vascularized by fenestrated capillaries which are devoided of blood brain barriers, these sites can thus be modulated either by circulating or locally-produced AII [13]. Subfornical organ and area prostrema contain a large number of AII receptors and are characterized by projections to numerous sites involved in the modulation of sympathetic discharges [14]. It is therefore possible that by its action on the subfornical organ and area prostrema, circulating AII could influence the sympathetic control of blood pressure and contribute to the resetting of the baroreflex sensitivity. It appears that the area prostrema may be an important site for the central modulation of ANS by circulating AII levels, since the ablation of this structure abolished the attenuating effect of AII on sensitivity of baroreflex and inhibited the increase in blood pressure associated with the chronic intravenous infusion of AII in the rat [15, 16]. This mechanism whereby AII acts directly on the baroreflex pathway may explain why the administration of AII increases blood pressure without being associated with a reflex bradycardia. During the long-term administration of AII, the initial rise in blood pressure would be due to a direct action on the vessels, whereas during the chronic phase of hypertension, the neurogenic effect of AII on the area prostrema would become dominant [17]. The importance of this latter mechanism in the development and maintenance of hypertension is suggested by the observation that the area prostrema of SHR contains a larger number of angiotensin receptors than that of their normotensive controls, thus suggesting that the attenuation of baroreflex-mediated sympathetic and heart rate responses by AII [18] may constitute an important mechanism of hypertension in that model.

Angiotensin II can also inhibit the central and peripheral vagal tone on the heart rate. Indeed, it was demonstrated, using the power spectral analysis of the variability of the heart rate, that the vagal tone was increased during the infusion of phenylephrine whereas the sympathetic modulation of the heart rate was enhanced during AII infusion in normal subjects [19]. Thus, the attenuation of the bradycardic response during angiotensin Infusion appears to be in great part due to the inhibition of the parasympathetic influence on the heart. In animal experiments whereby the vagus nerve activity was directly recorded, it was demonstrated that the increase in vagal nerve activity associated with an increase in blood pressure is significantly blunted during angiotensin Infusion thus confirming the central vagal inhibitory action of AII [20]. Moreover, an inhibitory action of AII on the peripheral vagus nerve has also been suggested by the observation of the bradycardic response induced by the stimulation of the vagus nerve [21]. These vagolitic actions of AII explain the increase in cardiac parasympathetic tone in heart failure patients during the treatment with ACEI [22, 23]. An important part of the beneficial effects of RAS blockers could thus result from their interactions with the activity of the central RAS. Although it was demonstrated that the chronic treatment with AT_1 receptor blockers reduces the blood pressure in association with the normalization of the sensitivity of the baroreflex response, it has not been clearly demonstrated whether the normalization of the baroreflex is directly linked to the blockade of central AT_1 receptors [23]. Several laboratories including our own have demonstrated the existence of an increased sympathetic tone and reactivity in an important proportion of the population of essential hypertensive patients, as well as in several models of experimental hypertension suggesting either a reduced sensitivity of the central baroreflex modulation of the sympathetic system or else, an increase in the sensitivity of facilitatory presynaptic receptors [1]. In hypertensive patients, we have demonstrated that the best responders to a therapy with ACEI were characterized by an increased sympathetic tone and reactivity before the initiation of the therapy and that the treatment attenuated the sympathetic reactivity to isometric exercise and to postural changes indicating an increase in the sensitivity of the baroreflex response [24]. Moreover, we have also demonstrated in one experimental model of hypertension (SHR), that the sympathetic response to the hypotensive action of sodium nitroprussiate was markedly attenuated by chronic treatments with either enalapril (ACEI) or losartan (AT_1 blocker), thus suggesting the restoration of the sensitivity of the baroreflex response under chronic RAS blockade [25]. In a recent study, Ligtenberg et al. [26] have clearly demonstrated in hypertensive patients with chronic renal disease, that the chronic treatment with ACEI not only restored the blood pressure, but also restored the sensitivity of the baroreflex response to changes in blood pressure as evaluated by the microneurographic recordings of muscle sympathetic fiber activity. This effect was specific to ACEI since the treatment with amlodipine also lowered the blood pressure, but failed to restore the baroreflex response. Similarly, the treatment of heart failure in patients with ACEI was also accompanied by a reduction in muscle sympathetic fiber activity [27]. It thus appears that the beneficial effects of RAS blockade in hypertension and heart failure could be due in great part to the sympatholytic effects of drugs inhibiting the activity of RAS. Those studies also suggest that the RAS may be implicated in the development of the sympathetic hyperactivity associated with hypertension and heart failure. This possibility also explains why patients with elevated sympathetic activity are better responders to this form of therapy. Moreover, the sympatholytic effects of those drugs would explain the absence of reflex tachycardia during the lowering of blood pressure induced by those agents.

Modulation of peripheral sympathetic nervous system by RAS

A significant contribution of specific cerebral structures has been suggested in the angiotensin-dependant control of autonomic function through central connection of the baroreflex arc [28]. Among others, the paraventricular, the parabrachial and the tractus solitarius nuclei show strong densities of angiotensin II receptors [29] in normotensive animals. These receptors are strongly enhanced in models with genetic hypertension. The renin-angiotensin pathway may also influence the parasympathetic system through the inhibition of vagal tone [30]. Consequently, in conditions of cardiac ischemia in which the renin angiotensin pathway is enhanced, heart rate and contractility may be abnormally increased.

On the other hand, it was demonstrated in several tissues in animal [31, 32], as well as in human atria [19] that AII potentiates the NE release from sympathetic nerve endings and catecholamine release from the adrenal medulla [33] by interacting with AT_1 receptors located on the presynaptic neuronal membrane or on the chromaffin cells presumably through the activation of protein kinase C. Furthermore, AII enhances the synthesis and reduces the neuronal uptake of catecholamines and will also potentiate the α_1 adrenergic receptor-dependant effects of noradrenalin. Considering that the sympathetic system also stimulates the secretion of renin through activation of the β_1 receptors localized in the kidney and blood vessels, one can suggest that there are reciprocal interactions between the two systems, as the activation of one would activate the other through positive retroactivity (Fig. 2). On the other hand, by blocking the effects of angiotensin II, one can attenuate the reactivity of the sympathetic system as well as its action on α_1 adrenergic receptors. These two latter properties will favor the restoration of α_1 adrenergic functions to normal, which will partly correct the sympathetic dysfunctions associated with essential hypertension [25].

Inhibition of the angiotensin converting enzyme significantly improves cardiopulmonary baroreflex control of sympathetic activity. Quinapril, through the inhibition of sympathetic nerve activity may, in part, contribute to the beneficial effects of ACE inhibitors on survival of patients with uncomplicated acute myocardial infarction [34]. Furthermore, other studies have shown a marked improvement in sympathetic and parasympathetic modulation of left ventricular systolic function with ACE inhibitor-treated patients during late morning and evening hours [35]. Hence, inhibition of ACE may be beneficial in the incidence of circadian pattern-dependent cardiac insults.

On the other hand, although the beneficial properties of ACE inhibitors are now clearly established [36], profound hypotension have been reported in chronically ACEI-treated patients under anesthesia [37, 38] in which the efficacy of α_1 adrenergic agonist is blunted [39, 40]. This particular hypotensive state has been suggested to be due to an imbalance of the sympathetic, renin-angiotensin and vasopressin systems in these patients [40]. In these situations, a vasopressin agonist, Terlipressin, has been shown to improve arterial pressure and increase vascular resistance in these patients [40]. The latter study clearly illustrates the promiscuous relation of the autonomic sympathetic, the renin angiotensin and vasopressin pathways.

Conclusion

This review illustrates the pivotal influence of the renin-angiotensin pathway on the autonomic nervous system and consequently on cardiovascular homeostasis. In cardiovascular diseases, the interaction between these two systems can be effectively interrupted through α or β blockade, ACE inhibition or AT_1 receptor blockade. On the other hand, there are no documented contributions of the AT_2 receptor in the modulation of the autonomic nervous system. Presence of AII, ACE and AT_1 receptors in the central nervous system and periphery strongly supports the important modulatory role of the angiotensin pathway on the central autonomic and peripheral nervous systems.

References

1 de Champlain J (1990) Pre- and postsynaptic adrenergic dysfunctions in hypertension. *J Hypertension* 8 (suppl 7): 577–585
2 Reid IA (1992) Interactions between Ang II, sympathetic nervous system, and baroreflexes in regulation of blood pressure. *Amer J Physiol* 262: E763–E778
3 Saxena PR (1992) Interaction between the renin-angiotensin-aldosterone and sympathetic nervous systems. *J Cardiovasc Pharmacol* 19 (suppl 6): S80–S86
4 Zanchetti AS (1977) Neural regulation of renin release: experimental-evidence and clinical implications in arterial-hypertension. *Circulation* 56: 691–698
5 Davis JO, Freeman RH (1976) Mechanisms regulating renin release. *Physiol Rev* 56: 1–56
6 Taddei S, Virdis A, Mattei P, Duranti P, Favilla S, Salvetti A (1994) Vascular renin-angiotensin system and sympathetic nervous system activity in human hypertension. *J Cardiovasc Pharmacol* 23: S9–S14
7 Bishop VS, Haywood JR (1991) Hormonal control of cardiovascular reflexes. *In*: IH Zucker, JP Gilmore (eds): *Reflex control of the circulation*. CRC, Boca Raton, FL, 1253–1271
8 Liard JF (1980) The baroreceptor reflexes in experimental hypertension. *Clin Exp Hypertension*

2: 479–498

9 Guo GB, Abboud FM (1984) Angiotensin II attenuates baroreceptor control of heart rate and sympathetic activity. *Amer J Physiol* 246: H80–H89

10 Goldsmith SR, Hasking GJ (1991) Effect of a pressor infusion of angiotensin II on sympathetic activity and heart rate in normal humans. *Circ Res* 68: 263–268

11 Kawano Y, Yoshida K, Matsuoka H, Omae T (1994) Chronic effects of central and systemic administration of losartan on blood pressure and baroreceptor reflex in spontaneously hypertensive rats. *Amer J Hypertens* 7: 536–542

12 Unger T, Badoer E, Ganten D, Lang RE, Rettig R (1998) Brain angiotensin: pathways and pharmacology. *Circulation* 77 (suppl 77): I40–I54

13 Ferguson AV, Bains JS (1997) Actions of angiotensin In the subfornical organ and area postrema: implications for long-term control of autonomic output. *Clin Exp Pharmacol Physiol* 24: 96–101

14 Matsukawa S, Reid IA (1990) Role of the area postrema in the modulation of the baroreflex control of heart rate by angiotensin II. *Circ Res* 67: 1462–1473

15 Fink GD, Bruner CA, Mangiapane MI (1987) Area postrema is critical for angiotensin-Induced hypertension in rats. *Hypertension* 9: 355–361

16 Cox BF, Bishop VS (1991) Neural and humoral mechanisms of angiotensin-dependent hypertension. *Amer J Physiol* 261: H1284–H1291

17 Andrews CO, Crim JW, Hartle DK (1993) Angiotensin II binding in area postrema and nucleus tractus solitarius of SHR and WKY rats. *Brain Res* 32: 419–424

18 Townend JN, Al-Ani M, West JN, Littler WA, Coote JH (1995) Modulation of cardiac autonomic control in humans by angiotensin II. *Hypertension* 25: 1270–1275

19 Lumbers ER, McCloskey DI, Potter EK (1979) Inhibition by angiotensin II of baroreceptor-evoked activity in cardiac vagal efferent nerves in the dog. *J Physiol-Lond* 294: 69–80

20 Potter EK (1982) Angiotensin Inhibits action of vagus nerve at the heart. *Brit J Pharmacol* 75: 9–11

21 Campbell BC, Sturani A, Reid JL (1985) Evidence of parasympathetic activity of the angiotensin converting enzyme inhibitor, captopril, in normotensive man. *Clin Sci* 68: 49–56

22 Osterziel KJ, Dietz R, Schmid W, Mikulatschek K, Manthey J, Kubler W (1990) ACE inhibition improves vagal reactivity in patients with heart failure. *Amer Heart J* 120: 1120–1129

23 Bartholomeusz B, Widdop RE (1995) Effect of acute and chronic treatment with the angiotensin II subtype 1 receptor antagonist EXP3174 on baroreflex function in conscious spontaneously hypertensive rats. *J Hypertension* 13: 219–225

24 de Champlain J, Yacine A, Leblanc R, Bouvier M, Lebeau R, Nadeau R (1994) Effects of trandolapril on the sympathetic tone and reactivity in systemic hypertension. *Amer J Cardiol* 73: 18C–25C

25 Laflamme AK, Oster L, Cardinal R, de Champlain J (1997) Effects of renin-angiotensin blockade on sympathetic reactivity and β-adrenergic pathway in the spontaneously hypertensive rat. *Hypertension* 30: 278–287

26 Ligtenberg G, Blankestijn PJ, Oey L, Klein IH, Dijkhorst-Oei LT, Boomsma F, Wieneke GH, van Huffelen AC, Koomans HA (1999) Reduction of sympathetic hyperactivity by enalapril in patients with chronic renal failure. *N Engl J Med* 340: 1321–1328

27 Grassi G, Cattaneo BM, Seravalle G, Lanfranchi A, Pozzi M, Morganti A, Carugo S, Mancia G (1997) Effects of chronic ACE inhibition on sympathetic nerve traffic and baroreflex control of circulation in heart failure. *Circulation* 96: 1173–1179

28 Phillips MI (1987) Functions of angiotensin In the central nervous system. *Annu Rev Physiol* 49: 413–435

29 Saavedra JM, Vishwanathan M, Shegmatsu K (1994) Characterisation and localization of angiotensin receptors in central and autonomic nervous systems regulating heart function. *In*: K Lindpainter, D Ganten (eds): *The cardiac renin angiotensin system*. Ganten, Armonk, NY, 125–139

30 Diz DI, Barnes KL, Ferrario CM (1986) Contribution of the vagus nerve to angiotensin II binding sites in the canine medulla. *Brain Res Bull* 17: 497–505

31 Zimmerman BG, Sybertz EJ, Wong PC (1984) Interaction between sympathetic and renin-angiotensin system. *J Hypertension* 2: 581–587

32 Story DF, Ziogas J (1987) Interaction of angiotensin with noradrenergic neuroeffector transmission. *Trends Pharmacol Sci* 8: 269–271

33 Wong PC, Hart SD, Zaspel AM, Chiu AT, Ardecky RJ, Smith RD, Timmermans PB (1990) Functional studies of nonpeptide angiotensin II receptor subtype-specific lignads: DuP 753 (AII-I)

and PD123177 (AII-2). *J Pharmacol Exp Ther* 255: 584–592

34 Hikosaka M, Yuasa F, Yuyama R et al. (2000) Effect of angiotensin-converting enzyme inhibitor on cardiopulmonary baroreflex sensitivity in patients with acute myocardial infarction. *Amer J Cardiol* 86: 1241–1244

35 Kontopoulos A, Athyros V, Papageorgiou A, Boudoulas H (1999) Effect of Quinapril or Metoprolol on circadian sympathetic and parasympathetic modulation after acute myocardial infarction. *Amer J Cardiol* 84: 1164–1169

36 The 1998 Joint National Committee (1998) The 1998 report of the Joint National Committee on detection, evaluation and treatment of high blood pressure. *Arch Intern Med* 148: 1023–1038

37 Colson P, Saussine M, Seguin JR, Cuchet D, Chaptal PA, Roquefeuil B (1992) Hemodynamic effects of anaesthesia in patients chronically treated with angiotensin-converting enzyme inhibitors. *Anesth Analg* 74: 805–808

38 Coriat P, Richer C, Douraki T, Gomez C, Hendricks K, Giudicelli JF, Viars P (1994) Influence of chronic angiotensin-converting enzyme inhibition on anesthetic induction. *Anesthesiology* 81: 299–307

39 Tuman KJ, McCarthy RJ, O'Connor CJ, Holm WE, Ivankovich AD (1995) Angiotensin-converting enzyme inhibitors increase vasoconstrictor requirements after cardiopulmonary bypass. *Anesth Analg* 80: 473–479

40 Licker M, Neidhart P, Lustenberger S, Valloton MB, Kalonji T, Fathi M, Morel DR (1996) Long-term angiotensin-converting enzyme inhibitors treatment attenuates adrenergic responsiveness without altering hemodynamic control in patients undergoing cardiac surgery. *Anesthesiology* 84: 789–800

41 Eyraud D, Brabant S, Dieudonne N, Nathalie D, Fleron MH, Gilles G, Bertrand M, Coriat P (1999) Treatment of intraoperative refractory hypotension with Terlipressin in patients chronically treated with an antagonist of the renin-angiotensin system. *Anesth Analg* 88: 980–984

Dual inhibitors of angiotensin converting enzyme and neutral endopeptidase

Cynthia A. Fink

Metabolic and Cardiovascular Diseases Research, Novartis, Biomedical Research Institute, Summit, New Jersey 07901, USA

Introduction

The development of single molecules which possess the ability to inhibit both angiotensin converting enzyme (EC 2.4.15.1, ACE) and neutral endopeptidase (EC 3.4.24.11, NEP) has been the recent focus of intensive drug discovery research [1, 2]. Both of these membrane-bound zinc metalloproteases are involved in the metabolism of peptides which modulate blood pressure and fluid homeostasis. ACE is part of the enzymatic cascade of the renin-angiotensin-aldosterone system and is largely responsible for the conversion of the biologically inactive decapeptide angiotensin-I to the octapeptide angiotensin-II. Angiotensin-II is a potent vasoconstrictor and triggers the release of the sodium retaining steroid aldosterone.

NEP is involved in the metabolic degradation of atrial natriuretic peptide (ANP) and is found in high concentrations in the brush border epithelial cells of the kidney and intestine [3, 4]. ANP is a 28 amino acid peptide which is secreted by the heart in response to atrial distension. Through interaction with its receptor, ANP induces an increase in c-GMP, which in turn elicits a number of biological responses including diuresis, natriuresis, vasodilation, and the inhibition of renin release and aldosterone biosynthesis [5, 6].

ACE inhibitors have gained wide acceptance clinically and have been prescribed for nearly two decades for the management of cardiovascular diseases. They are one of the most well tolerated class of therapeutic agents used for the treatment of hypertension and also have become a cornerstone for the treatment of congestive heart failure (CHF). The magnitude of blood pressure reduction that can be achieved with ACE inhibitor therapy is dependent on several factors, including the severity of hypertension, plasma renin activity, and the sodium status of the patient [7]. An adequate response with this therapy, however, is only achieved in about 50% of the essential hypertensive patient population, and it is most efficacious in individuals with high renin activity [8]. To increase the efficacy of this class of agents they can be co-administered with a diuretic [9]. Diuretics, however, can induce a number of undesired side effects including activation of pressor systems, hypokalemia, hyperglycemia, and elevation of plasma lipids [10]. Selective inhibitors of NEP have been shown to be effective in animal models of low renin activity and to produce diuresis with selective natriuresis in animals and humans [11]. Thus, there has been much interest in dual ACE and NEP inhibition as a potential new class of cardiovascular agents.

Rationale for dual ACE/NEP inhibition

Angiotensin-II and ANP act as functional antagonists at several cardiovascular target organs, and it is thus believed that potentiation of ANP with concurrent attenuation of angiotensin-II would produce additive and possibly synergistic beneficial effects in the control of fluid homeostasis and blood pressure regulation (Fig. 1). Several studies in animal models of hypertension and CHF have shown that coadministration of selective ACE and NEP inhibitors results in a potentiation of the effects produced by either agent alone [12, 13]. In addition, in a clinical study with essential hypertensive patients, it was observed that coadministration of sinorphan (NEP inhibitor) with captopril (ACE inhibitor) produced synergistic antihypertensive effects [14].

There have been several proposed explanations for the observed enhanced cardiovascular effects of dual inhibition. One hypothesis is that the decreased angiotensin II formation due to ACE inhibition may simply unmask the vasodilatory effects of endogenous ANP as well as other naturally occurring natriuretic peptides, such as brain natriuretic peptide (BNP) and C-type natriuretic peptide (CNP) [15]. In addition, BNP and CNP are substrates for NEP, thus a NEP inhibitor would protect them from degradation [16]. Bradykinin is also a substrate for both ACE and NEP, and thus inhibition of these enzymes might lead to a potentiation of this vasodilatory peptide [17]. In addition, ACE and NEP are able to metabolize substance P; therefore inhibitors of ACE and NEP may lead to a potentiation of this peptides vasodilatory activity [18].

Several selective inhibitors of NEP have been evaluated in clinical trials and were found to have little or no effect on blood pressure [1]. Interestingly, data from these clinical studies have revealed that there was an unexpected increase in angiotensin II levels in some patients [19, 20]. This would therefore limit the effectiveness of this class of drugs. The presence of an ACE inhibitor would block the formation of angiotensin II and thereby unmask the beneficial therapeutic effects of NEP inhibition leading to an enhancement in activity.

Single molecule dual ACE/NEP inhibitors

ACE and NEP are both membrane-bound proteases which from cloning and sequencing experiments, have been shown to belong to the thermolysin group of zinc-metalloproteases [11, 21]. These two enzymes possess similarities in

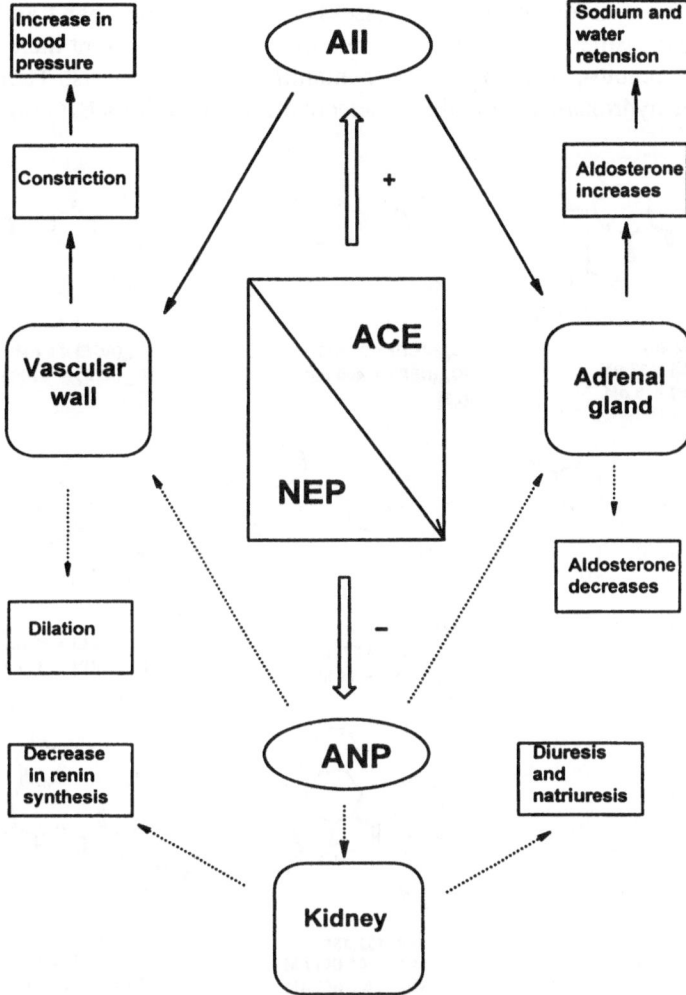

Figure 1. Functional effects of angiotensin-II and ANP.

their active sites, and their respective mechanisms of action. They also share common substrates. For example, both enzymes hydrolyze preferentially the Gly-Phe peptide bond of bradykinin and enkephalins *in vitro*.

As a result of the similarity between the two enzymes, rapid progress has been made in designing single molecules that have dual inhibitory activity. It is more desirable from developmental and clinical perspectives to have a single molecule which possess dual activity than attempting combination therapy. This will result in a more simple toxicology study and avoid more complicated pharmacokinetic issues arising from the administration of two molecules with different absorption and distribution properties. All of the single molecule dual inhibitors developed to date possess a zinc-chelating ligand and can be arbitrarily classified according to this binding group. At present there are car-boxyl-, mercapto-, and phosphoryl-containing dual inhibitors. There are a number of hydroxamate-containing selective NEP inhibitors but currently no

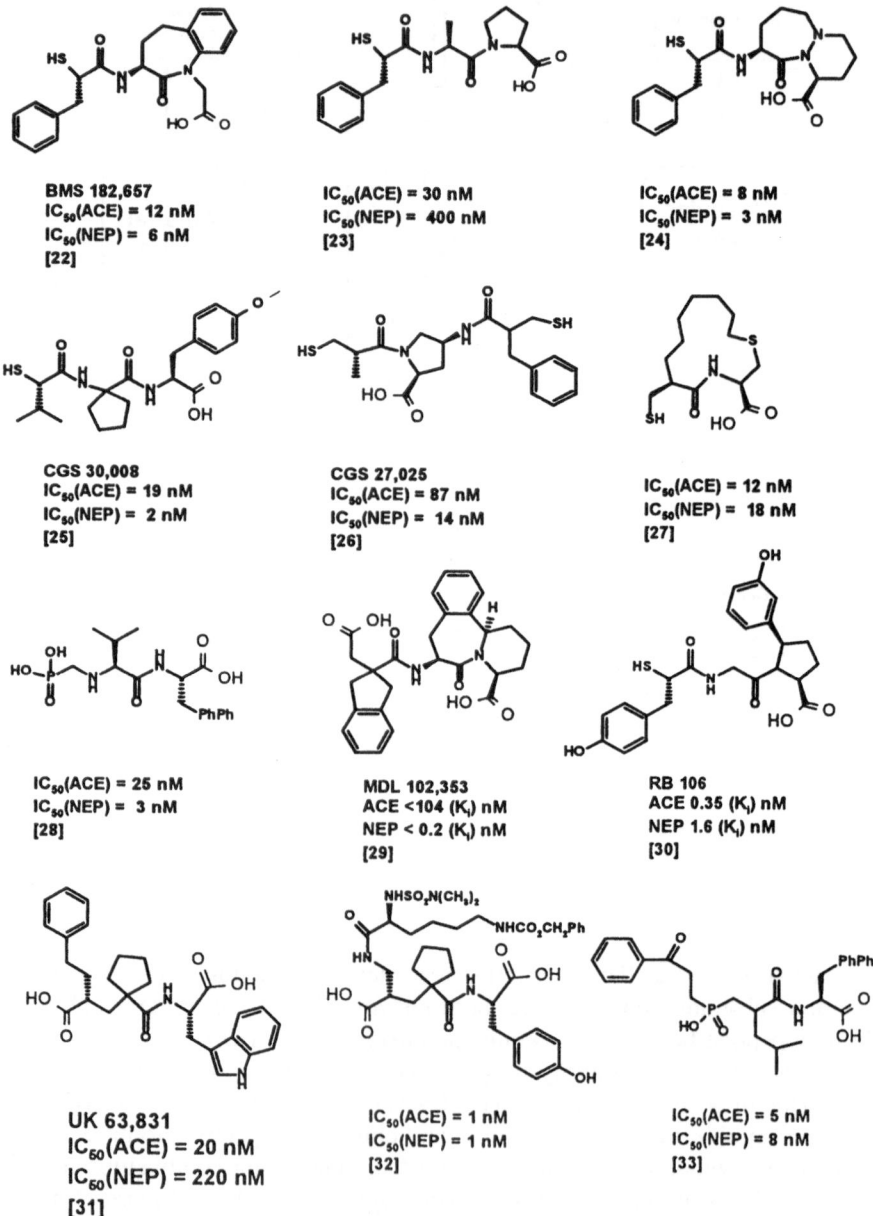

BMS 182,657
IC_{50}(ACE) = 12 nM
IC_{50}(NEP) = 6 nM
[22]

IC_{50}(ACE) = 30 nM
IC_{50}(NEP) = 400 nM
[23]

IC_{50}(ACE) = 8 nM
IC_{50}(NEP) = 3 nM
[24]

CGS 30,008
IC_{50}(ACE) = 19 nM
IC_{50}(NEP) = 2 nM
[25]

CGS 27,025
IC_{50}(ACE) = 87 nM
IC_{50}(NEP) = 14 nM
[26]

IC_{50}(ACE) = 12 nM
IC_{50}(NEP) = 18 nM
[27]

IC_{50}(ACE) = 25 nM
IC_{50}(NEP) = 3 nM
[28]

MDL 102,353
ACE <104 (K_i) nM
NEP < 0.2 (K_i) nM
[29]

RB 106
ACE 0.35 (K_i) nM
NEP 1.6 (K_i) nM
[30]

UK 63,831
IC_{50}(ACE) = 20 nM
IC_{50}(NEP) = 220 nM
[31]

IC_{50}(ACE) = 1 nM
IC_{50}(NEP) = 1 nM
[32]

IC_{50}(ACE) = 5 nM
IC_{50}(NEP) = 8 nM
[33]

Figure 2. Representative dual ACE/NEP inhibitors.

potent dual inhibitors from this class have been reported. Figure 2 shows representative dual ACE/NEP inhibitors reported in the literature. There are three published overviews on the design and pharmacology of dual inhibitors that should be reviewed for a more in-depth understanding of this field [1, 2, 7].

Dual inhibitors under clinical investigation

To date four dual ACE/NEP inhibitors have advanced into clinical trials. Three of these compounds are thiol-based inhibitors reported by workers at Bristol-Myers Squibb (BMS) [34], Hoechst Marion Roussel (HMR) [35], and Bioprojet [2]. A carboxylic acid dual inhibitor, sampatrilat (UK 81,252) was reported by workers at Pfizer [36]. The structures of these dual inhibitors is shown in Figure 3.

Currently the most advanced dual inhibitor is the BMS compound omapatrilat (BMS 186716). It is currently in phase III clinical studies for hypertension and phase II studies for congestive heart failure [37]. Omapatrilat is a potent inhibitor of ACE and NEP activity *in vitro*; with IC_{50} values of 5 and

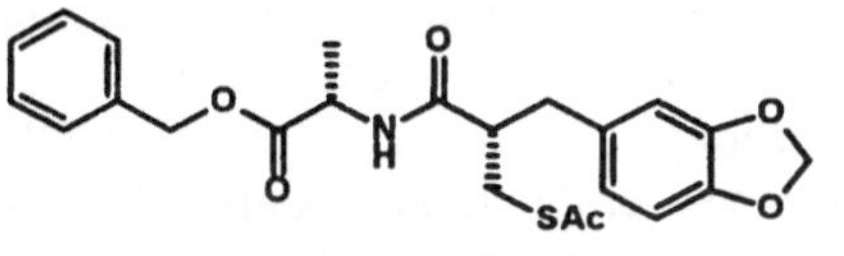

Aladotril
Phase II (France)
[2]

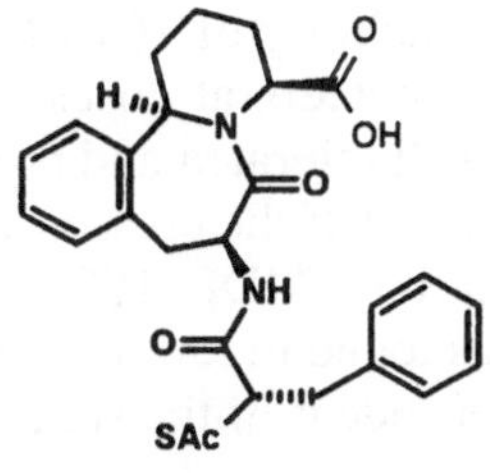

MDL 100, 240
Phase I
[35]

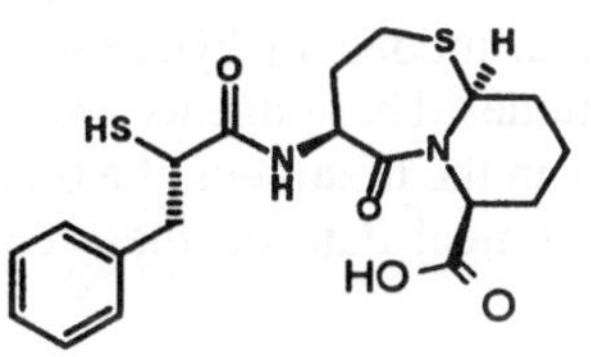

Omapatrilat
Phase III
[34]

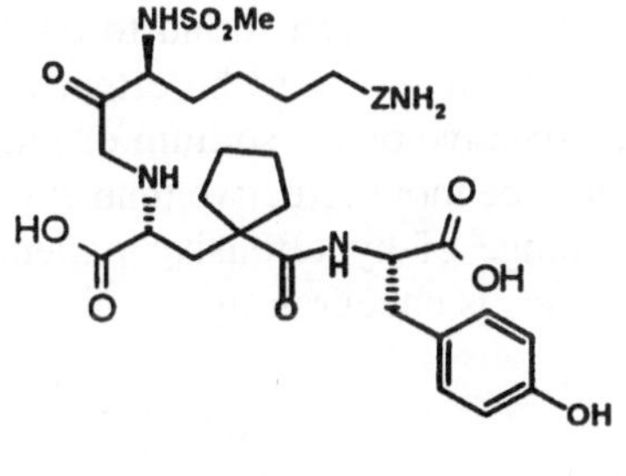

Sampatrilat
Phase II
[36]

Figure 3. Dual ACE/NEP inhibitors under clinical investigation.

8 nM respectively [34]. It has been found to be a long lasting, orally active antihypertensive agent in several different animal models of hypertension irrespective of the sodium or renin status of the model [38]. There has been one study reported in dogs examining the potential utility of this compound in the treatment of congestive heart failure [39]. Omapatrilat administered to dogs (10 mg/kg, po, BID) developing left ventricular failure by rapid pacing showed an improvement in myocyte basal contractility over control dogs. The limited clinical data that is available for this compound is also encouraging. Omapatrilat was administered to healthy males at doses ranging from 2.5 to 500 mg [40]. Mean arterial pressure was lowered by −4.6, −10, and −10.8 mmHg at the 2.5, 50, and 500 mg doses at 24 h. At all doses studied there was a decrease in plasma ACE activity that was still seen after 24 h. Also, an increase in the urinary excretion of cGMP was observed. The urinary excretion of ANP increased in a dose-dependent manner from 12.2 to 60 ng/day. Omapatrilat was well tolerated at doses up to 125 mg and side effects reported at the higher doses were headache, facial flushing, and nausea.

Information on the other dual ACE/NEP inhibitors under clinical evaluation is limited. Sampatrilat was administered to patients with essential hypertension (50 to 200 mg, po, single dose) and was found to lower blood pressure for at least 24 h [31]. The compound reportedly has a half-life of greater than 30 h with a bioavailability of 10%. MDL 100,240 was administered intravenously to healthy volunteers at doses ranging from 1.56 to 50 mg [35]. This compound was well tolerated and produced a dose-dependent inhibition of plasma ACE activity and of the pressor response to exogenous angiotensin I challenge. Like omapatrilat, MDL 100, 173 the carboxylic acid derivative of MDL 100,240, was found to lower blood pressure in several animal models of hypertension independent of the status of the plasma-renin activity [41].

Conclusion

Several ACE/NEP dual inhibitors have now been reported. Many of these compounds have been found to be potent dual inhibitors *in vitro* and in addition have been shown to be effective in different animal models of hypertension, irrespective of the sodium or renin status of the model. These agents possibly could be more effective than existing monotherapy in the treatment of a broader range of hypertensive patients. Thus far the clinical data on these compounds is encouraging.

References

1 De Lombaert S, Chatelain RE, Fink CA, Trapani AJ (1996) Design and pharmacology of dual angiotensin-converting enzyme and neutral endopeptidase inhibitors. *Curr Pharma Design* 2: 443–462

2 Fink CA (1996) Recent advances in the development of dual angiotensin-converting enzyme and neutral endopeptidase inhibitors. *Expert Opin Ther Patents* 6: 1147–1164; Robl JA, Ryono DE (1999) Recent advances in the design and development of vasopeptidase inhibitors. *Expert Opin Ther Patents* 9: 1665–1677

3 Kenny AJ, Stephenson SL (1988) Role of endopeptidase 24.11 in the inactivation of atrial natriuretic peptide. *FEBS Lett* 232: 1–8

4 Sonnenberg JL, Sakane Y, Jeng AY, Koehn JA, Ansell JA, Wennogle LP, Ghai RD (1988) Identification of protease NEP 24.11 as the major atrial natriuretic factor degrading enzyme in the rat kidney. *Peptides* 9: 173–180

5 Winquist RJ, Hintze TH (1990) Mechanism of atrial natriuretic factor-induced vasodilatation. *Pharmacol Ther* 48: 417–426

6 Johnson CI, Hodsman PG, Kohzuki M, Casley DJ, Fabris B, Phillips PA, Phil D (1989) Interaction between atrial natriuretic peptide and the renin angiotensin aldosterone system. *Amer J Med* 87: 24S–28S

7 Flynn GA, French JF, Dage RC (1995) Dual inhibitors of angiotensin converting enzyme and neutral endopeptidase: design and therapeutic rationale. *In*: JH Laragh, BM Brenner (eds): *Hypertension: pathophysiology, diagnosis, and management*. Raven Press, New York, 3099–3114

8 Laragh JH (1993) The renin system and new understanding of the complications of hypertension and their treatment. *Arzneim Forsch Drug Res* 43: 247–254

9 Townsend RR, Holland OB (1990) Combination of converting enzyme inhibitor with diuretic for the treatment of hypertension. *Arch Intern Med* 150: 1175–1183

10 Friedman PA (1988) Biochemistry and pharmacology of diuretics. *Semin Nephrol* 8: 198–212

11 Roques BP, Noble F, Dauge V, Fournie-Zaluski MC, Beaumont A (1993) Neutral endopeptidase 24.11 structure inhibition and experimental and clinical pharmacology. *Pharmacol Rev* 45: 87–146

12 Seymour AA, Asaad MM, Lanoce VM, Langenbacher KM, Fennell SA, Rogers WL (1993) Systemic hemodynamics, renal function and hormonal levels during inhibition of neutral endopeptidase 3.4.24.11 and angiotensin-converting enzyme in conscious dogs with pacing-induced heart failure. *J Pharmacol Exp Ther* 266: 872–883

13 Pham I, Gonzalez W, Amranni AI, Fournie-Zaluski MC, Philippe M, Laboulandine I, Roques BP, Michel JB (1993) Effects of converting enzyme inhibitor and neutral endopeptidase inhibitor on blood pressure and renal function in experimental hypertension. *J Pharmacol Exp Ther* 265: 1339–1347

14 Favrat B, Burnier M, Nussberger J, Lecomte JM, Brouard R, Waeber B, Brunner HR (1995) Neutral endopeptidase *versus* angiotensin converting enzyme inhibition in essential hypertension. *J Hypertension* 13: 797–804

15 Trippodo NC, Panchal BC, Fox M (1995) Repression of angiotensin II and potentiation of bradykinin contributute to the synergistic effects of dual metalloprotease inhibition in heart failure. *J Pharmacol Exp Ther* 272: 619–627

16 Kenny AJ, Bourne A, Ingram J (1993) Hydrolysis of human and pig brain natriuretic peptides, urodilatin, C-type natriuretic peptide and some C-receptor ligands by endopeptidase 24.11. *Biochem J* 291: 83–88

17 Skidgel RA (1992) Bradykinin-degrading enzymes: structure, function, distribution, and potential roles in cardiovascular pharmacology. *J Cardiovasc Pharm* 9 (suppl) S4–S9

18 Skidgel RA, Engelbrecht S, Johnson AR, Erdos EG (1984) Hydrolysis of substance P and neurotensin by converting enzyme and neutral endopeptidase. *Peptides* 5: 769–776

19 Richards AM, Wittert GA, Crozier IG, Espiner EA, Yandler TG, Ikram, H, Frampton C (1993) Chronic inhibition of endopeptidase 24.11 in essential hypertension: evidence for enhanced atrial natriuretic peptide and angiotensin II. *J Hypertension* 11: 407–416

20 Richards AM, Crozier IG, Kosaglou T, Rallings M, Espiner EA, Nicholls MG, Yandel TG, Ikram H, Frampton C (1993) Endopeptidase 24.11 inhibition by SCH 42495 in essential hypertension. *Hypertension* 22: 119–126

21 Wyvratt MJ, Patchett AA (1985) Recent developments in the design of angiotensin converting enzyme inhibitors. *Med Res* 5: 483–531

22 Robl JA, Simpkins LM, Stevenson J, Sun CQ, Murugesan N, Barrish JC, Asaad MM, Bird JE, Schaeffer TR, Trippodo NC, et al (1994) Dual metalloprotease inhibitors I. constrained peptidomimetics. *Bioorg Med Chem Lett* 4: 1789–1794

23 Delaney NG, Barrish JC, Neubeck R, Natarajan S, Cohen M, Rovnyak GC, Huber G, Murugesan

N, Girotra R (1994) Mercaptoacyl dipeptides as dual inhibitors of angiotensin converting enzyme and neutral endopeptidase. Preliminary structure activity studies. *Bioorg Med Chem Lett* 4: 1783–1788

24 Robl JA, Sun CQ, Simpkins LM, Ryono DE, Barrish JC, Karanewsky DS, Asaad MM, Schaeffer TR, Trippodo NC (1994) Dual metalloprotease inhibitors III. Utillization of bicyclic and monocyclic diazepinone bases mercaptoacyls. *Bioorg Med Chem Lett* 4: 2055–2060

25 Fink CA, Qiao Y, Berry CJ, Sakane Y, Ghai RD, Trapani AJ (1995) New alpha-thiol dipeptide dual inhibitors of angiotensin-I converting enzyme and neutral endopeptidase EC 3.4.24.11. *J Med Chem* 38: 5023–5030

26 Bhagwat SS, Fink CA, Gude C, Chan K, Qiao Y, Sakane Y, Berry C, Ghai RD (1994) 4-Substituted proline derivatives that inhibit angiotensin converting enzyme and neutral endopeptidase 24.11. *Bioorg Med Chem Lett* 4: 2673–2676

27 Stanton JL, Sperbeck DM, Trapani AJ, Cate D, Sakane Y, Berry CJ, Ghai RD (1993) Heterocyclic lactam derivatives as dual angiotensin converting enzyme and neutral endopeptidase 24.11 inhibitors. *J Med Chem* 36: 3829–3833

28 De Lombaert S, Tan J, Stamford L, Sakane Y, Berry C, Ghai RD (1994) Dual inhibition of neutral endopeptidase and angiotensin converting enzyme by N-phosphonomethyl and N-carboxy-alkyl dipeptides. *Bioorg Med Chem Lett* 4: 2715–2720

29 Merrel Dow Pharmaceuticals (1995) US 5,457,196

30 Fournie-Zaluski MC, Coric P, Thery V, Gonzalez W, Mendal H, Turcaud S, Michel JB, Roques BP (1996) Design of orally active dual inhibitors of neutral endopeptidase and angiotensin converting enzyme with long duration of action. *J Med Chem* 39: 2594–2608

31 James K (1995) Dual ACE/NEP inhibitors- from concept to clinic. *Eight RSC-SCI Med Chem Symp*, Cambridge, UK

32 Schering-Plough (1993) US 5,208,236

33 Zambon Group (1995) WO 9,535,302

34 Robl JA, Sun CQ, Stevenson J, Ryono DE, Simpkins LM, Cimarusti MP, Dejneka T, Slusarchyk WA, Chao S, Stratton L et al (1997) Dual metalloprotease inhibitors: mercaptoacetyl-based fused heterocyclic dipeptide mimetics as inhibitors of angiotensin-converting enzyme and neutral endopeptidase. *J Med Chem* 40: 1570–1577

35 Rousso P, Buclin T, Nussberger J, Brunner-Ferber F, Brunner HR, Biollaz J (1998) Effects of MDL 100,240, a dual inhibitor of angiotensin-converting enzyme and neutral endopeptidase on the vasopressor response to exogenous angiotensin I and angiotensin II challenges in healthy volunteers. *J Cardiovasc Pharmacol* 31: 408–417

36 Danser JAH (1995) Seventh European Meeting on Hypertension, June 9–12, Milan, Italy. *Expert Opin Invest Drugs* 4: 753–756

37 Fink CA (1998) Omapatrilat *IdDb* October

38 Trippodo NC, Robl JA, Asaad MM, Fox M, Panchal BC, Schaeffer TR (1998) Effects of omapatrilat in low, normal, and high renin experimental hypertension. *Amer J Hypertens* 11: 363–372

39 Thomas CV, McDaniel GM, Holzgrefe HH, Mukherjee RM, Hird RB, Walker JD, Hebbar L, Powell JR, Spinale FG (1998) Chronic dual inhibition of angiotensin-converting enzyme and neutral endopeptidase during the development of left ventricular dysfunction in dogs. *J Cardiovasc Pharmacol* 32: 902–912

40 BMS-186716 (1997) *Clinical Trials Monitor* 6: 13

41 French JF, Anderson BA, Downs TR, Dage RC (1995) Dual inhibition of angiotensin-converting enzyme and neutral endopeptidase in rats with hypertension. *J Cardiovasc Pharmacol* 26: 107–113

ACE Inhibitors
ed. by P. D'Orléans-Juste and G.E. Plante
© 2001 Birkhäuser Verlag/Switzerland

Pharmacodynamics, tissue-specificity of ACE inhibitors

Stylianos E. Orfanos[2], Linhua Zou[1] and John D. Catravas[1]

[1] Vascular Biology Center, Medical College of Georgia, Augusta, GA 30912-250, USA
[2] Department of Critical Care and Pulmonary Medicine, Evangelismos Hospital, University of Athens Medical School, Athens, Greece

Introduction

Angiotensin-converting enzyme (ACE) is a monomeric zinc dipeptidyl carboxypeptidase also known as kinase II. ACE is present as both a membrane-bound ectoenzyme and a soluble one. The former is found on endothelial cells, on absorptive epithelial and neuroepithelial cells, in the brain, and in the germinal cells of the testis. The latter is found in plasma and numerous other body fluids [1, 2]. ACE hydrolyzes the conversion of the decapeptide angiotensin I (Ang I) to the octapeptide angiotensin II (Ang II), as well as the degradation of the nonapeptide bradykinin [3]. Thus, ACE acts as a regulator between the renin-angiotensin and the kallikrein-kinin systems.

Renin-angiotensin system (RAS)

RAS plays a major role in increasing vascular tone, and regulating blood pressure, blood volume and electrolyte homeostasis in the circulation. Reduced sodium delivery at the macula densa, decreased renal perfusion pressure, and sympathetic activation will stimulate renin secretion by the juxtaglomerular cells of the afferent renal arterioles [3]. The aforementioned pathway is the classic source of renin in the circulating RAS, while renin may also be produced locally in tissues as part of the local, tissue-bound RAS. The former is expressed in many types of tissue, including the lungs, brain, kidneys, the vascular wall and cardiac muscle [4]. Renin cleaves the inactive decapeptide Ang I from the prohormone angiotensinogen; the former is then hydrolyzed by ACE to Ang II [3]. Ang II is a potent vasoconstrictor; it acts on vascular smooth muscle cells, interacts with the nervous system and causes volume expansion and fluid retention [2]. At the cellular level Ang II promotes migration, proliferation and hypertrophy [5, 6]. Most of these effects appear to be mediated through the AT_1 receptor, while the physiological significance of AT_2 receptors is still under investigation.

Kallikrein-kinin system

Plasma and tissue kallikreins are the main enzymes involved in the formation of kinins from kininogens. The arterial wall contains components of the kallikrein-bradykinin system. Bradykinin promotes, among others, vasodilation mainly through production of nitric oxide, arachidonic acid products and endothelium-derived hyperpolarizing factor [7]. In the kidneys, bradykinin causes natriuresis through direct tubular effects [2]. Most of these effects appear to be mediated through the B_2 receptor [8].

   ACE appears thus to regulate the balance between the vasodilatory properties of bradykinin and the vasoconstrictive properties of Ang II. Pharmacologically, the endothelium-bound/tisssue ACE rather than the serum ACE is mostly responsible for the aforementioned activity [9, 10] and appears to be the major site of action of ACE inhibitors.

ACE inhibitors

ACE inhibitors have been extensively studied and have been available for the treatment of hypertension for almost 20 years. More recent uses of ACE inhibitors however have included, among others, management of endothelial dysfunction (an early feature of coronary and systemic atherosclerosis), myocardial infarction, left heart hypertrophy and failure, and diabetic and collagen-disease related nephropathy [1, 11]. The need for longer-acting agents, in order to facilitate compliance, and agents with adequate pharmacokinetics and less adverse effects has led to the development of several ACE inhibitors [12].

Pharmacology

ACE inhibitors differ in the chemical structure of their active moiety, in potency, bioavailability, half-life, distribution, affinity for tissue bound ACE, and route of elimination [2]. They all have a common 2-methyl propranolol-L-proline moiety, that is important in blocking the active site of ACE [13]. ACE inhibitors may be classified in three groups, depending on their functional group that allows the adherence to the zinc component on the active site of ACE [11]: (i) sulfhydryl-containing, (ii) carboxyl-containing, and (iii) phosphinyl-containing group. Within each of these groups, there are significant differences in molecular weight and polarities. These differences have a significant influence on the routes of elimination and tissue distribution of the inhibitors. The latter, along with the intrinsic potency of a particular agent, will determine the magnitude of ACE inhibition at the tissue level [14].

   More than 14 ACE inhibitors are currently available worldwide; nine are available in the United States: captopril, enalapril, benazepril, lisinopril, moexipril, quinapril, ramipril, trandolapril and fosinopril. Captopril is the very first

ACE inhibitor to be used in clinical practice, and the prototype of the sulfhydryl-containing drugs [2]. Other inhibitors of this group are fentiapril, pivalopril, zofenopril and alacepril. Fosinopril is the only agent with a phosphinyl group, while the majority of all other agents contain a carboxyl moiety [2, 11]. Sulfhydryl-containing agents may have additional properties other than ACE inhibition. Several experimental studies have provided evidence that they act as free-radical scavengers and they attenuate nitrate tolerance [2, 11]. However, the clinical relevance of these observations has to be clarified further.

Captopril differs from all other agents due to its short half-life in plasma. Most ACE inhibitors are cleared predominantly by the kidney; trandolapril and fosinopril are additionally cleared by the liver [2]. The majority of these agents are administered as prodrugs, which are inactive until they are esterified in the liver. Captopril and lisinopril are the only oral agents that do not need hepatic activation to an active compound [11].

Tissue-specificity

There are substantial differences in the relative tissue affinity of ACE inhibitors. Part of these differences may be accounted for by the lipophilicity of each agent: high lipophilicity has been found to correlate with improved inhibition of local tissue enzyme in animal studies *in vivo* and *ex vivo* [11, 15]. In this respect trandolapril was superior to enalapril in inhibiting local tissue ACE activity in the heart, inner renal cortex, lungs aorta and adrenal glands [15]. Similar results were more recently obtained in our laboratory where treatment with trandolaprilat was found to be 5.5-, 3.6-, and 2.5-times more effective than enalaprilat in reducing ACE activities in rabbit aorta, left ventricle and lungs respectively [16]. Fabris and coworkers have examined the inhibition of ACE in the rat heart and found the order of inhibitor potency to be: quinalaprilat = benazaprilat > perindoprilat > lisinoprilat > fosinoprilat [17]. Quinapril was also more effective in preventing volume overload-induced ventricular hypertrophy in rats [18], while administration of enalapril and captopril in rats with heart failure revealed a stronger inhibitory action of enalapril on serum and lung ACE activities, a stronger inhibition of captopril on aortic ACE activity and comparable actions on renal ACE activity [19].

Assessment of endothelial-bound ACE activity *in vivo*

As already noted, endothelium-bound angiotensin converting ectoenzyme, and in particular pulmonary capillary endothelium-bound (PCEB) ACE appears to be the main locus where most of circulating Ang II synthesis and bradykinin break-down occur, probably because of the vast enzyme concentration and higher substrate availability in this vascular bed [12]. Therefore PCEB ACE should be the primary locus where ACE inhibitors exert their action and changes in PCEB ACE activity should closely relate to the major mechanism behind the obtained clinical antihypertensive effect [12, 16]. Consequently estimating PCEB ACE activity *in vivo* and the effects of ACE inhibitors administration on it, might provide accurate information on inhibitory potency and duration.

Applying indicator-dilution techniques, we and others have estimated PCEB-ACE activity in different models *in vivo*, by measuring the single pass transpulmonary hydrolysis, under first order reaction conditions, of synthetic substrates highly specific for ACE [1]. Endogenous substrates (Ang I, bradykinin) are not used in these kinds of studies, because they are also substrates for other naturally occurring enzymes. The most widely used synthetic substrate, so far, is benzoyl-Phe-Ala-Pro (BPAP), radiolabeled with ^{3}H [1]. Substrate hydrolysis is expressed as either %metabolism (%M), or v (=enzyme concentration $\times$ capillary transit time $\times$ k_{cat}/K_m), where k_{cat} is the catalytic rate constant and K_m is the Michaelis-Menten constant [20]. The modified kinetic parameter A_{max}/K_m (=enzyme mass $\times$ k_{cat}/K_m), an index of dynamically perfused capillary surface area may be additionally calculated [21]. Estimations of transpulmonary binding of radiolabeled ACE inhibitors have also been introduced [20].

Applications of PCEB ACE activity estimations for inhibition studies

Applying the aforementioned techniques we estimated BPAP transpulmonary metabolism (%) in rabbits immediately prior to, and 20 min post-iv administration of equiactive doses of either enalaprilat (10 µg/kg), or trandolaprilat (8 µg/kg). Both treatments decreased BPAP %M (Fig. 1a), with trandolaprilat causing a higher % decrease in BPAP %M (Fig. 1b). The more potent inhibition of PCEB ACE by trandolaprilat was maintained even when rabbits were co-treated with the calcium channel blocker verapamil [16]. Applying similar techniques, *in vivo*, may therefore provide quantifiable indices of PCEB ACE inhibition, allowing better evaluations of particular inhibitors.

Ryan and coworkers have recently shown that sequential PCEB ACE activity determinations, prior- and post-administration of an inhibitor, and the obtained hydrolysis (v) values, may be used to estimate the dissociation constant (k_{-1}) of the inhibitor enzyme reaction, *in vivo* [22]. We and others have provided evidence that trandolaprilat induces a longer lasting ACE inhibition than comparable doses of enalaprilat [12]. Consequently, we investigated if the longer inhibitory action of the former inhibitor was related to a longer lasting association with ACE, by administering the above-mentioned inhibitors in rabbits, with and without verapamil coadministration. Indeed, in our *in vivo* model, trandolaprilat exhibited $\approx$ threefold lower k_{-1} than enalaprilat; verapamil administration did not affect enalaprilat, but moderately increased the dissociation constant of trandolaprilat (Fig. 2) [12].

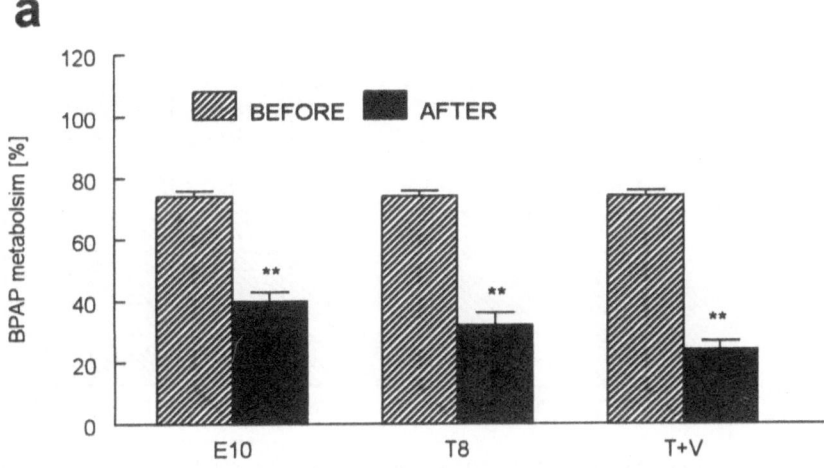

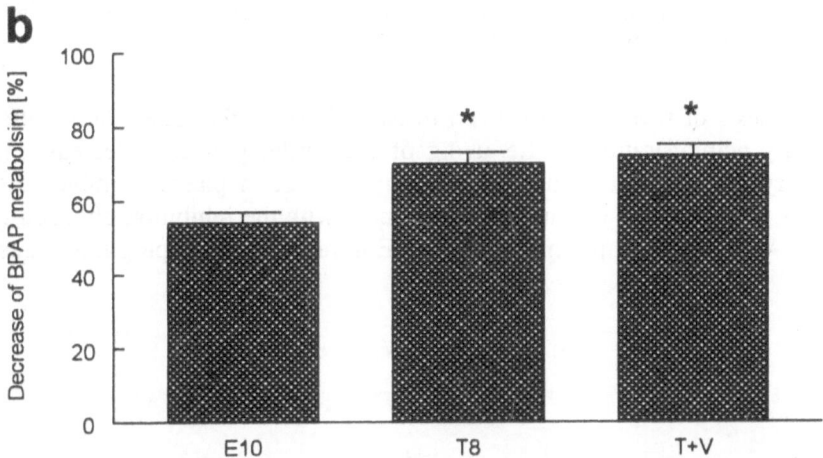

Figure 1. Effects of acutely administered ACE inhibitors on BPAP metabolism by PCEB ACE, *in vivo* (a), and corresponding percent inhibition of BPAP %M (b) Treatments: E10: 10 µg/kg enalaprilat; T8: 8µg/kg trandolaprilat; V: coadministration of 100 µg/kg verapamil. Means ± SE, [**]p < 0.01 from appropriate *BEFORE* values for panel a; [*]p < 0.05 from E10 values for panel b. (From [16], with permission).

Pulmonary endothelial ACE activity estimations in humans

The above-mentioned techniques have been recently introduced in humans [23, 24], providing evidence that they can be performed safely at the bedside, and establishing the range of PCEB ACE activity values for humans without lung disease [24]. More importantly, similar techniques were applied in the coronary circulation, a vascular bed where RAS may play a pivotal role in the

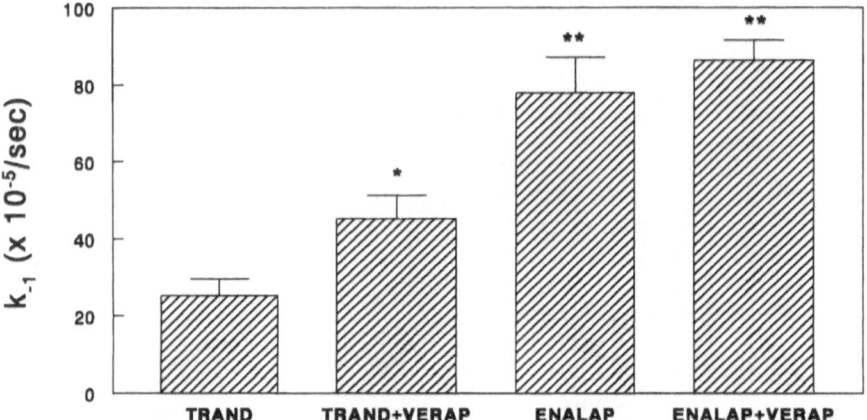

Figure 2. Dissociation constants $(k_{-1}) \times 10^{-5}/sec$ of trandolaprilat (TRAND) and enalaprilat (ENALAP), and when co-administered with verapamil (TRAND + VERAP) and (ENALAP + VERAP), from pulmonary capillary endothelium-bound ACE *in vivo*, applying the method of Ryan et al. [22]. Means ± SE, [*]$p < 0.05$ and [**]$p < 0.01$ from the k_{-1} of trandolaprilat with ANOVA and Dunnett's test (From [12], with permission).

pathogenesis of several severe heart diseases [23]. In the latter study, intra-coronary administration of 1.5 μg/kg of enalaprilat produced decreases in coronary endothelium-bound ACE activity but not in plasma soluble ACE activity (Fig. 3). This finding is in agreement with the inhibition obtained in PCEB ACE but not in plasma soluble ACE in rabbits, post captopril adminis-

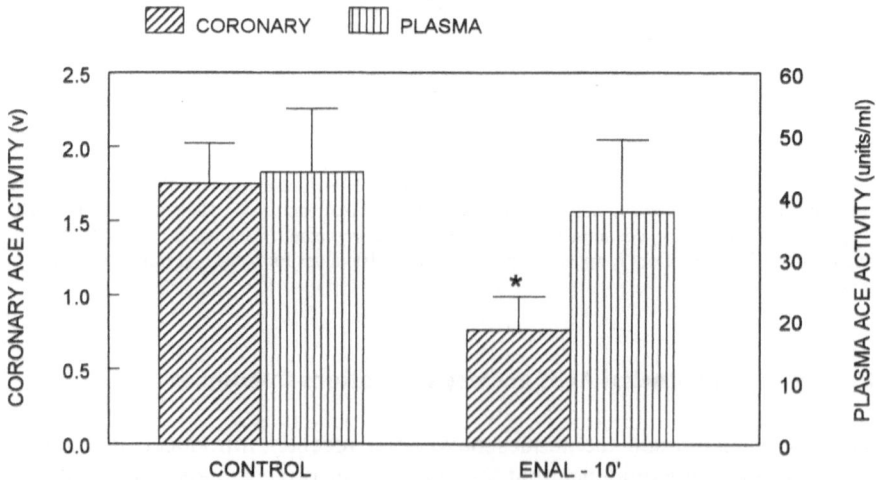

Figure 3. Coronary endothelium-bound vs plasma soluble ACE activity before and 10 min after enalaprilat administration in seven subjects undergoing elective coronary arterial bypass graft surgery. Means ± SE, [*]$p < 0.01$ from corresponding control (From [23], with permission).

tration [9], and might suggest a difference between mebrane-bound (endothelial) and soluble (plasma) ACE. Application of these techniques in humans appears to open a promising new frontier on ACE inhibitor research.

References

1 Catravas JD, Orfanos SE (1997) Pathopysiologic functions of endothelial angiotensin-converting enzyme. *In*: GVR Born, CJ Schawtz (eds): *Vascular Endothelium. Physiology, Pathology and Therapeutic Opportunities*. Schattauer, Stuttgart, 193–204

2 Brown NJ, Vaughan DE (1998) Angiotensin-converting enzyme inhibitors. *Circulation* 97: 1411–1420

3 Jackson EK, Garisson JC (1996) Renin and angiotensin. *In*: JG Hardman, LE Limbird (eds): *Goodman's and Gilman's The Pharmacological Basis of Therapeutics (9th edition)*. McGraw-Hill, New York, 733–758

4 Bastien N, Lambert C (1998) Effect of treatment on survival in an animal model of chronic heart failure. *Amer J Cardiol* 82 (10A): 50S–52S

5 Bell L, Madri J (1990) Influence of the angiotensin system on endothelial and smooth muscle cell migration. *Amer J Pathol* 137: 7–12

6 Daemen MJ, Lombardi DM, Bosman FT, Schwartz SM (1991) Angiotensin II induces smooth muscle cell proliferation in the normal and injured rat arterial wall. *Circ Res* 68: 450–456

7 Vanhoutte PM (1998) Endothelial dysfunction and inhibition of converting enzyme. *Eur Heart J* 19 (suppl J): J7–J15

8 Regoli D, Barabe J (1980) Pharmacology of bradykinin and related kinins. *Pharmacol Rev* 32: 1–46

9 Chen I, Pitt BR, Moalli R, Gillis CN (1984) Correlation between lung and plasma angiotensin converting enzyme and the hypotensive effect of captopril in conscious rabbits. *J Pharmacol Exp Ther* 229: 649–653

10 Esther CR, Marino EM, Howard TE (1997) The critical role of tissue angiotensin-converting enzyme as revealed by gene targeting in mice. *J Clin Invest* 99: 2375–2385

11 White CM (1998) Pharmacologic, pharmacokinetic and therapeutic differences among ACE inhibitors. *Pharmacotherapy* 18 (3): 588–599

12 Orfanos SE, Parkerson J, Fisher E, Catravas JD (1998) Estimation of the dissociation constants for pulmonary endothelial angiotensin-converting enzyme reactions with trandolaprilat and enalaprilat *in vivo*. *Drug Dev Res* 44: 80–86

13 Williams GH (1988) Converting enzyme inhibitors in the treatment of hypertension. *N Engl J Med* 319: 1517–1525

14 Ondetti MA (1988) Structural relationships of angiotensin converting- enzyme inhibitors to pharmacologic activity. *Circulation* 77 (suppl I): I74–I78

15 Wiserman LR, McTavish D (1994) Trandolapril: a review of its pharmacodynamic and pharmacokinetic properties, and therapeutic use in essential hypertension. *Drugs* 48: 72–90

16 Cziraki A, Parkerson J, Fisher E, Catravas JD (1997) Inhibition of pulmonary endothelial angiotensin converting enzyme activity by trandolaprilat *in vivo*. *Drug Dev Res* 41: 22–30

17 Fabris B, Jackson B, Cubela R, Mendelsohn FAO, Johnston CI (1989) Angiotensin converting enzyme in the rat heart: studies of its inhibition *in vitro* and *ex vivo*. *Clin Exp Pharmacol Physiol* 16: 309–313

18 Ruzicka M, Skarda V, Leenan FHH (1995) Effects of ACE inhibitors on circulating *versus* cardiac angiotensin II in volume overload-induced cardiac hypertrophy in rats. *Circulation* 92: 3568–3573

19 Hirsch AT, Talsness CE, Smith AD, Schunkert H, Ingelfinger JR, Dzau VJ (1992) Differential effects of captopril and enalapril on tissue renin-angiotensin systems in experimental heart failure. *Circulation* 86: 1566–1574

20 Ryan JW, Catravas JD (1991) Angiotensin converting enzyme as an indicator of pulmonary microvascular function. *In*: MA Hollinger (ed.): *Focus on Pulmonary Pharmacology and Toxicology*. CRC Press, Boca Raton, 183–210

21 Catravas JD, White RE (1984) Kinetics of pulmonary angiotensin-converting enzyme and 5'-nucleotidase *in vivo*. *J Appl Physiol* 57: 1173–1181

22 Ryan JW, Falido MJ, Sequeira MJ, Chung AYK, Berryer P, Chen XL, Catravas JD (1994) Estimation of rate constants for reactions of pulmonary microvascular angiotensin converting enzyme with an inhibitor and a substrate *in vivo*. *J Pharmacol Exp Ther* 270: 260–268
23 Douraki T, Theodoropoulos S, Catravas JD (1995) Measurement of enalaprilat-induced inhibition of coronary endothelium-bound angiotensin converting enzyme activity in patients undergoing coronary arterial bypass graft surgery. *In*: Ch Roussos et al. (ed.): *8th European congress of intensive care medicine*. Monduzzi Editore, Bologna, 527–531
24 Orfanos SE, Langleben D, Khoury J, Schlesinger RD, Dragatakis L, Roussos Ch Ryan JW, Catravas JD (1999) Pulmonary capillary endothelium-bound angiotensin converting enzyme activity in humans. *Circulation* 99: 1593–1599

ACE Inhibitors
ed. by P. D'Orléans-Juste and G.E. Plante
© 2001 Birkhäuser Verlag/Switzerland

Effect of angiotensin converting enzyme inhibition on thirst and salt-appetite

Tewfik Nawar, Eve-Reine Gagné, Raymonde Turcotte and Gérard E. Plante

Departments of Medicine (Nephrology), Physiology and Pharmacology, Institute of Pharmacology, University of Sherbrooke, Sherbrooke (Québec) Canada

Introduction

Normally, eating and drinking provide the body with a surplus of water and electrolytes. Water and sodium balance therefore are normally achieved by renal regulation. Stimulation of water and salt intake are back-up mechanisms [1].

Thirst is the perception of a need for water. This sensation is relieved by drinking water. Increased sodium appetite results from a need for sodium. This sensation is relieved by consuming salt. Salt hunger is well-known in the animal kingdom [2]. As early as 1884, Manley wrote: "the universal existence of an appetite for salt surely indicates that the substance serves more important functions than that of merely gratifying the palate" [3].

Homeostasis of fluid and electrolytes is most important. More than a century ago, Claude Bernard described the constancy of the "milieu intérieur". Plasma osmolality is normally maintained within a very narrow range. Variations of only 1 to 2% initiate mechanisms to return the plasma osmolality to normal. Effective circulating volume (defined as the extracellular fluid which is in the arterial system and is effectively perfusing the tissues) is also extremely important, and its control is complex involving multiple sensors and effectors [4, 5]. Mechanisms for preservation and restoration of circulatory volume are essential. Hypovolemia elicits a reflex response of the heart and blood vessels followed by mobilisation of interstitial fluid. When hypovolemia becomes persistent or severe, thirst and sodium appetite are stimulated [1].

Angiotensin-II and thirst

An increase in serum osmolality is the main stimulus for vasopressin release and thirst. The concept of hypothalamic osmoreceptors originally described by Verney is now well accepted although questions remain concerning the precise location of such receptors and their relation to possible sodium sensitive receptors.

Another dipsogenic agent is angiotensin-II. This peptide induces a vigorous short-latency burst of drinking. This is one of the most striking stimulatory effects of any substance on any motivated behaviour [1].

The effect of angiotensin-II on drinking is most obvious after intracranial administration. After intracranial injection in a rat, the animal stops whatever it is doing and starts to drink, usually less than one minute after the injection. Drinking is usually completed within 15 min. After a large dose of angiotensin-II, the amount of water drunk is comparable to the 24-h intake of water of a normal rat [6].

An increase in drinking can also be produced by systemic administration of angiotensin-II. However, this effect is more variable and sometimes absent probably because the dipsogenic action of angiotensin-II is opposed by inhibitory discharge from cardiovascular stress receptors responding to the pressor effect of systemic angiotensin-II.

The dipsogenic effect of angiotensin-II is found in most mammals and birds. This widespread occurrence in phylogeny reflects the evolutionary importance of defending the circulation [1]. Angiotensin-II is the major mediator of hypovolemic thirst. The threshold blood loss for stimulating hypovolemic thirst is 8–10% (compared to 1–2% loss of all water for osmotic thirst) [1–7]. Interestingly, this is also the threshold for non-osmotic stimulation of vasopressin release.

Despite its powerful dipsogenic action delineation of the precise role of angiotensin-II in physiological thirst has been difficult to demonstrate.

All the known effects of the angiotensin-II on cardiac contractility, vasoconstriction, vascular hypertrophy, renal hemodynamics, release of aldosterone and vasopressin as well as the action on the brain are mediated by AT_1 receptors. AT_2 receptors are highly expressed in the foetus and also in the adult in certain pathological conditions [8–10]. Their exact function is not clear, but AT_1/AT_2 receptors may have opposing effects on several physiological responses and possibly on drinking behaviour. AT_2 receptors could also have a role in the long-term organisation of drinking [1].

Angiotensin-II and salt appetite

The effect of angiotensin-II on sodium intake is more complex and more difficult to study. In contrast to its effect on water intake, intracranial angiotensin-II induces a slowly developing and persistent increase in sodium intake [11]. This suggests that angiotensin-II is doing more than simply stimulating the appropriate neurons [1]. Among other actions, angiotensin-II affects protein synthesis, cell growth, membrane function, learning and memory, all of which could be involved in the development of sodium appetite. Angiotensin-II induced increased sodium intake complements the renal sodium retaining action of angiotensin-II. The effects of angiotensin-II on salt appetite is also mediated by the AT-1 receptors. There are data suggesting that AT_2 receptors could have a permissive role in salt appetite. The effects of systemic angiotensin-II infusion are inconsistent and more difficult to evaluate because of concomitant mineralocorticoid secretion (which independently could stimulate sodium appetite) and because of possible interference due to angiotensin-II pressor effects.

The influence of angiotensin-II on sodium intake was more difficult to demonstrate than its dipsogenic effect. However, its physiological role is more convincingly demonstrated.

Role of brain angiotensin peptides

The classic renin-angiotensin system consists of renin produced by the kidney, renin substrate (angiotensinogen) produced by the liver and angiotensin converting enzyme localized in the vasculature and the lungs. There is now ample evidence that angiotensin-II can also be generated locally (independent of circulating renin) in many tissues including the brain [12], arteries, ventricles, adrenal glands, kidneys, ovaries, testis, uterus and others. In many cases, the actions of these local tissue systems complement those of circulating angiotensin-II.

Angiotensin-II does not penetrate easily the blood brain barrier. Some of the angiotensin-II sensitive neurons are accessible to circulating angiotensin-II, these include the circumventricular organs (CVO) which lack the blood brain barrier [13]. Three of the CVO, the subformical organ (SFO), organum vasculosum of the lamina terminalis (COVLT) and the area postrema, contain neurons responsive to angiotensin-II. Other angiotensin sensitive structures involved in thirst and sodium appetite lie inside the blood brain barrier and cannot be reached directly by circulating angiotensin-II. Most brain nuclei for which an effect of angiotensin-II has been demonstrated contain AT_1 receptors. These receptors have been mapped in the central nervous system of a number of species (including man). The distribution of AT_1 receptors is highly conserved across mammalian species.

There are uncertainties about the function of brain angiotensin peptides and their relation to circulating angiotensin-II. It is believed, however, that angiotensin peptides of central origin may contribute to increased thirst caused by dehydration and to the increased sodium appetite due to sodium depletion. A significant hypovolemia is a threat to life and therefore elicits a coordinated response designed to restore the circulating volume. Angiotensin-II, both circulating and central, is an important component of that response.

Angiotensin-II can therefore be viewed as one of the major mechanisms helping to maintain effective circulating blood volume and is particularly important in hypovolemia. The effects of angiotensin-II in water and Na intake complement its well-known vasoconstrictive and renal sodium retaining effects.

It should be remembered, however, that most of the reported experimental observations have been made in rats. It is not known if all these findings apply to man.

Effect of angiotensin converting enzyme inhibitors

The effect of angiotensin converting enzyme (ACE) inhibitors on thirst and sodium appetite depends on the dose, route of administration, duration of treatment and presence of external stimuli to thirst and sodium intake. These experiments are complicated by the fact that various other biologically active peptides (bradykinin, substance-P, neurokinin, neurotensin, and others) are normally cleaved by ACE and will therefore be affected by ACE inhibitors.

ACE inhibition decreases circulating angiotensin-II. This results in an increased renal renin secretion (which is normally inhibited by angiotensin-II) and there is therefore also an increase in circulating angiotensin-I. In the brain, the increased amount of blood-borne angiotensin-I could be converted to angiotensin-II by unblocked ACE (especially if ACE-inhibitors do not easily cross the blood brain barrier, for example: quinapril and benazapril). Furthermore, angiotensin-II can be produced by non-ACE pathways.

Effect of ACE inhibition on thirst and sodium appetite

Experimental observations

Systemic administration of ACE-inhibitors increases water intake. A review of the extensive literature on this subject [1] shows that this dipsogenic effect has the following convincing characteristics. (1) It is absent in nephrectomized animals. (2) It is abolished by intracranial administration of ACE-inhibitors indicating that it depends on locally-produced angiotensin-II. (3) It is increased in rats with bilateral ureteral ligation indicating that the effect is not related to urine flow. Interestingly, in these animals, enhanced water intake occurs despite the increasing water retention. (4) It is abolished if renin secretion is suppressed by mineralocorticoids.

Therefore, the dipsogenic effect of ACE-inhibitors is due to an increase in renal renin secretion and depends on the presence of enough unblocked ACE (or other enzymes) in the brain to convert increased angiotensin-I to angiotensin-II. This effect is more powerful in conditions where there is an increased baseline renin secretion.

The effect of ACE inhibition on sodium appetite is less consistent and depends on the experimental model. In general, the following results have been repeatedly reported in short-term and long-term experiments. (a) Short-term administration of low doses of ACE inhibitors increases sodium intake under conditions where there is a previous chronic activation of the renal renin angiotensin system (for example in adrenalectomized rats). No effect was observed in DOCA-treated rats on a high salt diet where renal renin production is inhibited. However, following short-term administration of high doses of ACE-inhibitors, there is a decrease in sodium intake in rats with renin-dependent enhanced sodium intake (for example in sodium depleted animals). (b) In contrast, the long-term administration of ACE-inhibitors to normal rats induces a slow and progressive increase in sodium intake.

Clinical observations

The effect of ACE inhibitors on salt appetite in human subjects has not been explored to our knowledge, yet anecdotal reports in hypertensive patients treated with captopril suggest that the weight gain and elevation of blood pressure which develops on occasion and reponds to addition of hydrochlorothiazide, could be related to enhanced sodium intake due to alteration in salt appetite [14]. We therefore examined the effect of two ACE inhibitors, captopril and perindopril, on salt appetite in 21 mild to moderate hypertensive patients with normal renal function. The results indicate that the threshold for sodium chloride detection increased significantly from 31 to 50 mM, and from 28 to 56 mM, respectively, after two and four weeks of therapy. However, the hedonic counterpart of the salt detection threshold, examined with the sodium chloride preference test, indicated that lower concentrations of sodium chloride solutions, 34 and 36 mM, for captopril and perindopril, respectively, were chosen by both groups of patients tested in a blind fashion. The latter findings were confirmed by the fact that urinary sodium excretion values were not different following ACE inhibition therapy, and the body weight of patients remaining unchanged as well [15].

The mechanisms responsible for the observed adjustment of salt appetite, as reflected by the preference test, could involve down-regulation of the receptors located in the oral mucosa, as described for other tissues, and/or adaptation of the hypothalamic center involved in the control of sodium appetite. The clinical significance of these findings will obviously require further studies.

References

1 Fitzsimons JT (1998) Angiotensin, thirst and sodium appetite. *Physiol Rev* 78: 583–686
2 Denton DA (1982) *The hunger for salt*. Springer Verlag, Berlin
3 Ritz E (1996) The history of salt – aspects of interest to the nephrologist. *Nephrol Dialysis Transplant* 11: 969–975
4 Gauer OH, Henry JP (1963) Circulatory basis of fluid volume control. *Physiol Rev* 43: 423–481
5 Schrier RW (1992) A unifying hypothesis of body fluid regulation. *J Roy Coll Physician Lond* 26: 295–306
6 Epstein AN, Fitzsimons JT, Rolls BJ (1970) Drinking induced by infusion of angiotensin Into brain of the rat. *J Physiol* 210: 457–474

7 Fitzsimons JT (1961) Drinking by rats depleted of body fluid without increase in osmotic pressure. *J Physiol* 159: 297–309

8 Unger T, Chung T, Csikos T et al (1996) Angiotensin receptors. *J Hypertension* 14 (suppl 5): S95–S103

9 Allen AM, Moeller I, Jenkins TA (1998) Angiotensin receptors in the nervous system. *Brain Res* 47: 17–28

10 Inigami T (1999) Molecular biology and signaling of angiotensin receptors: an overview. *J Amer Soc Nephrol* 10: S2–S7

11 Blair-West JR, Carey KD, Denton DA (1998) Evidence that brain angiotensin II is involved in both thirst and sodium appetite in baboons. *Amer J Physiol* 275: R1639–1646

12 Ganten D, Unger T, Lang T (1988) The brain renin-angiotensin system: basic and functional considerations. *In*: JW Harding, JW Wright, RC Speth, CD Barnes (eds): *Angiotensin and Blood Pressure*. Academic Press, San Diego, 117–133

13 McKinley MJ, McAllen RM, Mendelsohn FAO (1990) Circumventricular organs: neuroendocrine interfaces between the brain and hemal milieu. *Frontiers Neuroendocrinol* 11: 91–127

14 Turcotte R, Lussier Y, Plante GE (1987) L'appétit pour le sodium. *Médecine Sci* 3: 33A

15 Plante GE, Gagné ER, Turcotte R (1993) Converting enzyme inhibition and salt appetite. *In*: JB Puschett, A Greenberg (eds): *Diuretics IV: Chemistry, Pharmacology and Clinical Applications*. Elsevier Science Publishers, Amsterdam, 609–612

ACE Inhibitors
ed. by P. D'Orléans-Juste and G.E. Plante
© 2001 Birkhäuser Verlag/Switzerland

ACE and diabetes

Mark E. Cooper

Department of Medicine, University of Melbourne, Austin and Repatriation Medical Centre (Repatriation Campus), West Heidelberg, Victoria 3081, Australia

Diabetic vascular complications

Diabetes is associated with both micro and macrovascular complications. The predominant microvascular disorders are retinopathy, nephropathy and neuropathy whereas macrovascular disease affects, from a clinical point of view, mainly the coronary, peripheral and cerebrovascular trees [1]. The major cause of death in diabetes is atherosclerotic vascular disease but microvascular disease remains an important cause of morbidity in the diabetic population [1]. Diabetic renal disease is the major cause of end stage renal failure in the western world and proliferative retinopathy and maculopathy remain common causes of blindness in the world. Any strategy that can retard, reverse or prevent any of these diabetic complications would be of major benefit to the diabetic population.

The renin-angiotensin system in diabetes

Initially, it was viewed that the renin-angiotensin system (RAS) was suppressed in diabetes. Such an opinion was based on plasma measurements of various components of the RAS including plasma renin activity and angiotensin II (AII) concentrations [2]. However, over the last 15 years it has become increasingly apparent that there is a local renin-angiotensin system at sites of vascular injury. These sites include not only the kidney but also the blood vessel wall [3] and more recently the retina [4]. Using molecular biological and immunohistochemical techniques investigators have reported normal, increased and decreased levels of various components of the RAS in the kidney in experimental diabetes. More recently, our group has measured by sensitive radioimmunoassay the levels of the various angiotensin peptides in the diabetic kidney and as suggested previously there was no evidence in whole kidney that angiotensin levels are increased in experimental diabetes [5]. However, the kidney is a heterogeneous organ and using techniques which explore the distribution of renin and angiotensin II it has been shown in other models of renal injury that despite suppression of the systemic RAS within the kidney and in particular in damaged proximal tubules there is aberrant expression of renin and AII which could subsequently lead to elaboration of prosclerotic cytokines resulting in progressive renal fibrosis [6]. Pilot studies by our group suggest that such a phenomenon is also occurring in experimental diabetes and complements studies by Anderson et al. suggesting local activation of the RAS in diabetes [7]. Recent *in vitro* studies in a proximal cell line have suggested that glucose *per se* promotes angiotensinogen expression providing a mechanism linking metabolic to vasoactive hormone pathways in diabetes [8]. Not only is there evidence of activation of the RAS by glucose at the cellular level but studies exploring the mechanisms whereby glucose and vasoactive hormones such as AII mediate vascular injury in diabetes have suggested several sites where the pathways may interact [9]. For example, AII and glucose activate protein kinase C, an intracellular second messenger which has been implicated in the pathogenesis of diabetic complications [9]. A number of vascular growth factors have been identified which have proliferative and prosclerotic actions relevant to the pathological processes involved in diabetic vascular disease. These include transforming growth factor-β (TGF-β) and vascular endothelial growth factor (VEGF) which have been shown to be both glucose and AII dependent [9]. Although this review focuses on the RAS, other vasoactive hormones including both vasoconstrictors and vasodilators have been postulated to play a role in mediating diabetic vascular complications [10]. The role of these hormones is of increasing interest with the advent of inhibitors of these peptides providing an option for new therapeutic approaches for diabetic complications.

AII, the effector molecule of the RAS, has multiple actions relevant to the pathogenesis of diabetic complications. This hormone not only elevates systemic blood pressure, a major accelerating factor for diabetic complications but has important effects on intrarenal hemodynamics including preferential effects on efferent arteriolar resistance, elevation of intraglomerular pressure, effects on mesangial cell contraction and glomerular permselectivity and stimulation of proximal tubular ion transport [11]. In addition, AII is a potent angiogenic peptide relevant to the pathogenesis of diabetic retinopathy and has prosclerotic actions relevant to extracellular matrix accumulation, a process associated with basement membrane thickening and the development of glomerulosclerosis.

Experimental studies

The landmark studies by Brenner's group suggested that ACE inhibitors could confer a renoprotective role in normotensive diabetic rats [11]. Micropuncture studies suggested that this renoprotection was mediated via effects on intrarenal hemodynamics including reduction in intraglomerular pressure [11]. More recent studies by our group have suggested that although hemodynamic factors may play a pivotal role in mediating the beneficial effects of ACE inhibitors in the diabetic kidney, this probably involves suppression of TGFβ-dependent pathways in both the glomerulus and the tubulointerstitium [12]. Further studies have been performed comparing other antihypertensive agents to ACE inhibitors. Dihydropyridine calcium antagonists, despite similar reductions in blood pressure, were not as effective as ACE inhibitors in preventing renal injury in both hypertensive and normotensive diabetic rats [13, 14].

Our group has also explored the role of ACE inhibitors in preventing diabetes-associated vascular hypertrophy in the mesenteric vascular tree in experimental diabetes. ACE inhibition reduced the wall/lumen ratio, a measure of vascular hypertrophy [15]. These effects were associated with less endothelial proliferation, less matrix accumulation in both the medial and adventitial layers and reduced gene expression of both TGFβ and the matrix protein, type IV collagen [15]. Similarly designed studies are now in progress to assess the role of ACE inhibition in preventing retinopathy.

Clinical studies

Before the onset of microalbuminuria, blood pressure is already increasing but hypertension, as conventionally defined, is not usually apparent until overt proteinuria develops. Numerous studies have shown that control of systemic hypertension has a major effect on reducing proteinuria and slowing progression to renal failure in both type I and type II diabetes [16].

ACE inhibitors in diabetic renal disease

Normoalbuminuria

The observation that ACE inhibitors slow progression in microalbuminuric type I diabetic patients [17] has led to consideration that it may be of benefit in diabetic patients prior to the development of microalbuminuria. However, in the EUCLID study, no evidence for a beneficial role for the ACE inhibitor, lisinopril, was observed in normoalbuminuric type I diabetic subjects, despite evidence that it reduced the development of retinopathy [18]. However, the lack of an observed effect may have been related to the short duration of only two years for the study. Ravid et al. have addressed whether ACE inhibitors provide protection in normotensive, normoalbuminuric type II diabetic subjects [19]. These investigators suggested that treatment in this population retarded the development of microalbuminuria. However, a significant proportion of type II diabetic subjects are hypertensive at presentation with hypertension being one of the components of the insulin resistance syndrome [20].

Microalbuminuria associated with normal BP

The exciting observation by Brenner's group that ACE inhibitors lower glomerular pressure and prevent glomerular damage in diabetic rats independent of effects on systemic hypertension [11] led to a large number of clinical studies to explore the role of ACE inhibition in normotensive type 1 diabetic patients with early renal disease [17]. These studies have clearly documented that ACE inhibitors will decrease microalbuminuria and retard the development of frank proteinuria in type I diabetes. However, it is not always clear whether the effect is independent of blood pressure (BP) in these studies, as most cases involved comparing ACE inhibitors to placebo, and as a consequence systemic BP was often lower in the ACE treated groups.

The effect of ACE inhibitors on progression in normotensive microalbuminuric type II diabetic subjects has also been studied. Although many type II diabetic patients with microalbuminuria are hypertensive, a significant proportion will be normotensive (BP < 140/90 mmHg), particularly in the Asian population. Studies comparing ACE inhibitors to placebo have also suggested a benefit, particularly in decreasing the risk for developing proteinuria [17]. In the study by Ravid et al., treatment with enalapril for five years was not only associated with a reduced risk for developing proteinuria, but was also associated with stabilization of renal function. In contrast, the placebo treated group had a 13% decline in renal function [21]. Similar findings have been reported by several other investigators in Indo-Asian populations. Whether or not these findings can be extrapolated to type II diabetic subjects in other racial groups will have to await further studies.

Microalbuminuric or proteinuric patients with hypertension

Most studies have shown that ACE inhibitors can reduce proteinuria of any aetiology [22]. A range of studies have documented that ACE inhibitors will more effectively reduce proteinuria in either type I or type II diabetic subjects when compared with standard antihypertensive therapy using diuretics and β-blockers [23]. In addition to reducing proteinuria, ACE inhibitors may slow the deterioration of renal function. For example, in the Collaborative Study, captopril treatment was compared to placebo in type I diabetic subjects with proteinuria and mildly impaired renal function [24]. Treatment was associated with a slowing of the deterioration of renal function over the three-year period [24].

In type II diabetic subjects with microalbuminuria and hypertension, ACE inhibitors have also been shown to be more potent at reducing proteinuria than conventional therapy (diuretic and β blockers) [17]. It is less evident whether ACE inhibitors are superior to other antihypertensive agents in type II diabetic subjects with albuminuria, although in general most studies have shown some advantage to either ACE inhibitors or nondihydropyridine calcium channel blockers (such as diltiazem or verapamil) particularly when compared to dihydropyridine calcium channel blockers (CCBs) in reducing proteinuria and stabilizing renal function [25].

While the above studies clearly document the benefit of ACE inhibitors in normotensive and hypertensive microalbuminuric patients with type I and, to a lesser extent, type II diabetes, it is still unclear if the mechanism is independent of their BP lowering effects. For example, in the Collaborative Study there was clearly less benefit in type I diabetic subjects with normal BP and relatively preserved renal function. A recent meta-analysis also could not show superiority of ACE inhibitors over other agents at maximum hypotensive doses [26]. The concept of focusing on aggressive BP reduction rather than ACE inhibition *per se* is further suggested by a recent study by the Collaborative Study group. Proteinuric type I diabetic subjects received either low or high dose ramipril. Patients on high dose had a BP that was 7 mmHg lower with a reduction in albuminuria whereas the low dose group had an increase in albuminuria [27]. This study was unable to discern if the superior efficacy of the high dose ramipril group was related to lower blood pressure or more effective blockade of the RAS.

Experimental studies suggest that AT1 receptor antagonists may have similar beneficial effects to ACE inhibitors in diabetic renal disease [28]. Studies are now being completed and analyzed to address the role of this new class of drugs in diabetic renal disease [29].

ACE inhibitors and cardioprotection

The choice of antihypertensive therapy in the diabetic population needs to be considered in the context of not only providing renoprotection but also the potential effects of these agents on atherosclerotic events. Indeed, diabetic patients with persistent microalbuminuria are at increased risk for all-cause mortality, especially from cardiovascular disease. Therefore, the monitoring of other cardiovascular risk factors in these patients is critical. Several studies suggest that ACE inhibitors may provide additional cardioprotective effects in hypertensive patients with either type I or type II diabetes. In the GISSI-3 trial, lisinopril treatment was associated with improved 30-day survival in diabetic patients after an acute myocardial infarct [30]. In the ABCD trial, in which cardiovascular endpoints were assessed, the hypertensive arm of the study was prematurely halted due to a possible superiority of the ACE inhibitor over the calcium channel antagonist in terms of cardiovascular events [31]. In the FACET study involving 380 hypertensive type II diabetic subjects it was also shown that the ACE inhibitor, fosinopril, was associated with less cardiovascular events than amlodipine [32]. In the recent HOT study which involved felodipine-based antihypertensive treatment, aggressive blood pressure reduction in the diabetic subgroup was associated with reduced cardiovascular mortality [33]. However, in that study the group with the lowest tertile of blood pressure had the highest prevalence of concomitant therapies including ACE inhibitors. Therefore, it remains to be determined if the improved cardiovascular outcome in the diabetic population with the lowest blood pressure levels was due to effective blood pressure reduction or to a specific vasoprotective effect of ACE inhibition. In the CAPPP trial, an advantage of the ACE inhibitor over conventional therapy (diuretics, β blockers) was observed in the diabetic subgroup [34]. By contrast, in the United Kingdom Prospective Diabetes Study (UKPDS), both captopril and atenolol were associated with reduced cardiovascular events without evidence that one agent conferred a specific additional benefit [35]. It is anticipated that over the next few years results from other studies will become available which include larger numbers of diabetic patients as well as subjects treated with AII receptor antagonists. Indeed, several multicenter studies are currently examining the effects of AT1 receptor antagonists on both renal and cardiovascular endpoints in type 2 diabetic patients.

Retinopathy

Angiotensin II has angiogenic properties and therefore it is possible that this hormone may play a role in mediating neovascularisation in the diabetic retina. Although this possibility has not been extensively investigated, in the EUCLID study which evaluated the role of lisinopril in a population of predominantly normotensive, normoalbuminuric type I diabetic subjects, ACE inhibition was associated with at least a 50% reduction in retinopathy including proliferative retinopathy [36]. This issue requires further investigation since this study provides preliminary evidence for a retinoprotective role for agents which interrupt the RAS.

Guidelines for treatment in the diabetic population

The Sixth Joint National Committee (JNC-VI) has recommended a relatively aggressive approach to treating hypertension in the diabetic population [37]. It was suggested that treatment be considered at a BP of 130/85 with a goal BP of 125/75 in proteinuric patients. These guidelines extend recommendations from other organisations who have also suggested more aggressive BP targets in the diabetic population [38]. ACE inhibitors are the preferred choice as first line treatment in diabetic patients with hypertension and/or renal disease by some of these organisations but this is not a universal recommendation.

In summary, AII has pleiotropic actions relevant to the pathogenesis of diabetic complications. A large number of clinical studies have confirmed a major role for ACE inhibitors in diabetic nephropathy. There is increasing evidence for a vasoprotective role for these agents and preliminary data suggest a potential beneficial effect in diabetic retinopathy.

References

1 Clark CJ, Lee DA (1995) Prevention and treatment of the complications of diabetes mellitus. *N Engl J Med* 332: 1210–1217
2 Allen TJ, Cooper ME, O'Brien RC, Bach LA, Jackson B, Jerums G (1990) Glomerular filtration rate in the streptozocin diabetic rat: The role of exchangeable sodium, vasoactive hormones and insulin therapy. *Diabetes* 38: 1182–1190
3 Dzau V (1988) Circulating *versus* local renin-angiotensin system in cardiovascular homeostasis. *Circulation* 77 (suppl 1): 1–4
4 Berka JL, Stubbs AJ, Wang DZM, Di Nicolantonio R, Akorn D, Campbell DJ, Skinner SL (1995) Renin containing Müller cells of the retina display endocrine features. *Invest Ophthalmol Visual Sci* 36: 1450–1458
5 Campbell DJ, Kelly DJ, Wilkinson-Berka JL, Cooper ME, Skinner SL (1999) Increased bradykinin and 'normal' angiotensin peptide levels in streptozotocin-diabetic Sprague Dawley and TGR(mRen-2) rats. *Kidney Int* 71: 211–221
6 Gilbert RE, Wu LL, Kelly DJ, Cox A, Wilkinson-Berka JL, Johnston CI, Cooper ME (1999) Pathological expression of renin and angiotensin II in the renal tubule following subtotal nephrectomy: implications for the pathogenesis of tubulointerstitial fibrosis. *Amer J Pathol* 155: 429–440
7 Anderson S, Jung FF, Ingelfinger JR (1993) Renal renin-angiotensin system in diabetes: functional, immunohistochemical, and molecular biological correlations. *Amer J Physiol* 265: F477–F486
8 Zhang SL, Filep JG, Hohman TC, Tang SS, Ingelfinger JR, Chan JSD (1999) Molecular mechanisms of glucose action on angiotensinogen gene expression in rat proximal tubular cells. *Kidney Int* 55: 454–464
9 Cooper ME (1998) Pathogenesis, prevention and treatment of diabetic nephropathy. *Lancet* 352: 213–219
10 Tikkanen T, Tikkanen I, Rockell MD, Allen TJ, Johnston CI, Cooper ME, Burrell LM (1998) Dual inhibition of neutral endopeptidase and angiotensin-converting enzyme in rats with hypertension and diabetes mellitus. *Hypertension* 32: 778–785
11 Zatz R, Dunn BR, Meyer TW, Brenner B (1986) Prevention of diabetic glomerulopathy by pharmacological amelioration of glomerular capillary hypertension. *J Clin Invest* 77: 1925–1930
12 Gilbert RE, Cox A, Wu LL, Allen TJ, Hulthen UL, Jerums G, Copper ME (1998) Expression of transforming growth factor-β1 and type IV collagen in the renal tubulointerstitium in experimental diabetes: effects of angiotensin converting enzyme inhibition. *Diabetes* 47: 414–422
13 Anderson S, Rennke HG, Brenner BM (1992) Nifedipine *versus* fosinopril in uninephrectomized diabetic rats. *Kidney Int* 41: 891–897
14 Rumble JR, Doyle AE, Cooper ME (1995) Comparison of effects of ACE inhibition with calcium channel blockade on renal disease in a model combining genetic hypertension with diabetes. *Amer J Hypertens* 8: 53–57
15 Rumble JR, Gilbert RE, Cox A, Wu L, Cooper ME (1998) Angiotensin converting enzyme inhibition reduces the expression of transforming growth factor-beta(1) and type IV collagen in diabetic vasculopathy. *J Hypertension* 16: 1603–1609
16 Parving H-H, Andersen AR, Smidt VM, Hommel E, Mathiesen ER, Svendsen PA (1987) Effect of antihypertensive treatment on kidney function in diabetic nephropathy. *Brit Med J* 294: 1443–1447
17 Cooper ME (1996) Renal protection and ACE inhibition In microalbuminuric type I and type II diabetic patients. *J Hypertension* 14 (suppl 6): S11–S14
18 The EUCLID study group (1997) Randomised placebo-controlled trial of lisinopril in normotensive patients with insulin-dependent diabetes and normoalbuminuria or microalbuminuria. *Lancet* 349: 1787–1792
19 Ravid M, Brosh D, Levi Z, Bardayan Y, Ravid D, Rachmani R (1998) Use of enalapril to attenuate decline in renal function in normotensive, normoalbuminuric patients with type 2 diabetes mellitus – a randomized, controlled trial. *Ann Intern Med* 128: 982–988
20 Williams B (1994) Insulin resistance: the shape of things to come. *Lancet* 344: 521–524
21 Ravid M, Savin H, Jutrin I, Bental T, Katz B, Lishner M (1993) Long-term stabilizing effect of angiotensin-converting enzyme inhibition on plasma creatinine and on proteinuria in normotensive type II diabetic patients. *Ann Intern Med* 118: 577–581
22 Ruggenenti P, Perna A, Mosconi L, Matalone M, Garni G, Salvadori M, Zoccali C, Scolari F,

Maggiore Q, Tognoni et al (1997) Randomised placebo-controlled trial of effect of ramipril on decline in glomerular filtration rate and risk of terminal renal failure in proteinuric, non-diabetic nephropathy. *Lancet* 349: 1857–1863

23 Kasiske BL, Kalil RS, Ma JZ, Liao M, Keane WF (1993) Effect of antihypertensive therapy on the kidney in patients with diabetes: a meta-regression analysis. *Ann Intern Med* 118: 129–138

24 Lewis EJ, Hunsicker LG, Bain RP, Rohde RD (1993) The effect of angiotensin converting enzyme inhibition on diabetic nephropathy. *N Engl J Med* 329: 1456–1462

25 Bakris GL, Copley JB, Vicknair N, Sadler R, Leurgans S (1996) Calcium channel blockers *versus* other antihypertensive therapies on progression of NIDDM associated nephropathy. *Kidney Int* 50: 1641–1650

26 Weidmann P, Schneider M, Bohlen L (1995) Therapeutic efficacy of different antihypertensive drugs in human diabetic nephropathy: an updated meta-analysis. *Nephrol Dialysis Transplant* 10 (suppl): 39–45

27 Lewis EJ, Rohde R, Bain R, for the Collaborative Study Group (1997) A follow-up study of the course of nephropathy in type I diabetes mellitus. *Nephrology* 3 (suppl 1): P1222

28 Allen TJ, Cao Z, Youssef S, Hulthen UL, Cooper ME (1997) The role of angiotensin II and bradykinin in experimental diabetic nephropathy: functional and structural studies. *Diabetes* 46: 1612–1618

29 Rodby RA (1997) Antihypertensive treatment in nephropathy of type II diabetes: role of the pharmacological blockade of the renin-angiotensin system. *Nephrol Dialysis Transplant* 12: 1095–1096

30 Zuanetti G, Latini R, Maggioni AP, Franzosi M, Santoro L, Tognoni G (1997) Effect of the ACE inhibitor lisinopril on mortality in diabetic patients with acute myocardial infarction – data from the GISSI-3 study. *Circulation* 96: 4239–4245

31 Estacio RO, Jeffers BW, Hiatt WR, Biggerstaff SL, Gifford N, Schrier RW (1998) The effect of nisoldipine as compared with enalapril on cardiovascular outcomes in patients with non-insulin-dependent diabetes and hypertension. *N Engl J Med* 338: 645–652

32 Tatti P, Pahor M, Byington RP, Di Mauro P, Guarisco R, Strollo G, Strollo F (1998) Outcome results of the Fosinopril *versus* Amlodipine Cardiovascular Events randomised Trial (FACET) in patients with hypertension and non-insulin dependent diabetes mellitus. *Diabetes Care* 21: 597–603

33 Hansson L, Zanchetti A, Carruthers SG, Dahlof B, Elmfeldt D, Julius S, Menard J, Rahn KH, Wedel H, Westerling S (1998) Effects of intensive blood-pressure lowering and low-dose aspirin in patients with hypertension: principal results of the Hypertension Optimal treatment (HOT) randomised trial. *Lancet* 351: 1755–1762

34 Hansson L, Lindholm LH, Niskanen L, Lanke J, Hedner T, Niklason A, Luomanmati K, Dahlof B, de Faire U, Morlin C et al (1999) Effect of angiotensin-converting-enzyme inhibition compared with conventional therapy on cardiovascular morbidity and mortality in hypertension: the Captopril Prevention Project (CAPPP) randomised trial. *Item Corporate Author CAPPP study grp* 353: 611–616

35 Stearne MR, Palmer SL, Hammersley MS, Franklin SL, Spivey RS, Levy JC, Tidy CR, Bell NJ, Steemson J (1998) Efficacy of atenolol and captopril in reducing risk of macrovascular and microvascular complications in type 2 diabetes – UKPDS 39. *Brit Med J* 317: 713–720

36 Chaturvedi N, Sjolie A-K, Stephenson JM, Abrahamian H, Keipes M, Castellarin A, Rogulja-Pepeonik Z, Fuller JH (1998) Effect of lisinopril on progression of retinopathy in people with type 1 diabetes. *Lancet* 351: 28–31

37 Joint National Committee on Prevention Detection Evaluation, Treatment of High Blood Pressure (1997) The sixth report of the Joint National Committee on Prevention, Detection, Evaluation, and Treatment of High Blood Pressure. *Arch Intern Med* 157: 2413–2445

38 Mogensen CE, Keane WF, Bennett PH, Jerums G, Parving HH, Passa P, Steffes MW, Striker GE, Viberti GC (1995) Prevention of diabetic renal disease with special reference to microalbuminuria. *Lancet* 346: 1080–1084

Subject index